Amblyopia: A Multidisciplinary Approach

Publisher: Caroline Makepeace
Development editor: Robert Edwards
Production Controller: Chris Jarvis
Desk editor: Claire Hutchins
Cover designer: Greg Harris

Amblyopia: A Multidisciplinary Approach

edited by

Merrick Moseley

Senior Lecturer, Imperial College of Science, Technology and Medicine, London, UK

Alistair Fielder

Kennerley Bankes Professor of Ophthalmology, Imperial College of Science, Technology and Medicine, London, UK

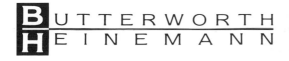

BUTTERWORTH
HEINEMANN

OXFORD AUCKLAND BOSTON JOHANNESBURG MELBOURNE NEW DELHI

Butterworth-Heinemann
Linacre House, Jordan Hill, Oxford OX2 8DP
225 Wildwood Avenue, Woburn, MA 01801–2041
A division of Reed Educational and Professional Publishing Ltd

℞ A member of the Reed Elsevier plc group

First published 2002

British Library Cataloguing in Publication Data
Amblyopia: a multidisciplinary approach
  1. Amblyopia   2. Amblyopia – Diagnosis   3. Amblyopia – Treatment
  4. Pediatric ophthalmology
  I. Moseley, Merrick   II. Fielder, Alistair R.
  617.7'62

Library of Congress Cataloguing in Publication Data
A catalogue record for this book is available from the Library of Congress

ISBN 0 7506 4691 8

For information on all Butterworth-Heinemann publications visit our website at
www.bh.com

Composition by Genesis Typesetting, Laser Quay, Rochester, Kent
Printed and bound in Great Britain by the Bath Press, Avon

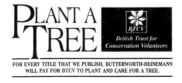

FOR EVERY TITLE THAT WE PUBLISH, BUTTERWORTH-HEINEMANN
WILL PAY FOR BTCV TO PLANT AND CARE FOR A TREE.

Contents

Contributors

Stephen J. Anderson

The Wellcome Trust Laboratory for MEG Studies, Neurosciences Research Institute, Aston University, Birmingham, UK

Alistair Fielder

Faculty of Medicine, Imperial College of Science, Technology and Medicine, London, UK

Robert F. Hess

McGill Vision Research, Department of Ophthalmology, McGill University, Montreal, Quebec, Canada

Lynne Kiorpes

Center for Neural Science, New York University, USA

Merrick Moseley

Faculty of Medicine, Imperial College of Science, Technology and Medicine, London, UK

Barnaby C. Reeves

Health Services Research Unit, London School of Hygiene and Tropical Medicine, London, UK

Preface

The origins of this book stem from a conversation held between us some five years ago, in which we pondered the many different approaches taken to unravel this enigmatic condition. In some areas, principally in the basic sciences, progress in the latter twentieth century appeared to be gathering momentum, whereas in others, notably in the more applied areas, progress appeared to be faltering. Perhaps such an observation could just as equally be applied to the study of so many other clinical conditions, yet what struck us in particular about amblyopia was how little interchange of ideas occurred between the various subdisciplines; put in colloquial terms, little appeared to be trickling down from laboratory to clinic, *or indeed to be trickling up from clinic to laboratory.* Such a state of affairs is undoubtedly inimical to progress, and prompted us to organize, in January 1999, a small gathering of researchers under the auspices of the Novartis Foundation. At this meeting, held in London, progress in key subdisciplines was reviewed, including those of sensory processing in humans and animals, functional neuroimaging, epidemiology, treatment and disability. Subsequently, individuals who took a leading role in this meeting were asked to update and commit their subject reviews to paper, and this monograph is principally the product of their endeavours. We have also included here the transcript of the discussion component of the Novartis Foundation meeting, which gives a more intimate insight into the concerns of those currently working in this area. Debate was lively – in some cases passionate and heated – but importantly, we would hope, particularly insightful for those entering this area of research.

We proudly hope that what is included here, appearing as it does shortly after the beginning of the new millennium, may, with the passage of time, be considered a benchmark by which progress in amblyopia research, be it slow or rapid, will come to be judged.

Merrick Moseley

Alistair Fielder

Acknowledgements

The editors gratefully acknowledge the support of the Novartis Foundation.

Cover illustration courtesy of Kris Singh and Stephen Anderson.

1 Sensory processing: animal models of amblyopia

Lynne Kiorpes

INTRODUCTION

Wiesel and Hubel launched an era of intense research with their Nobel Prize-winning studies on the effects of visual experience on the development of the visual system. Beginning in the early 1960s, they characterized the functional organization of the primary visual cortex and discovered the vulnerability of this organization to abnormal visual experience in early postnatal life (Wiesel and Hubel, 1963, 1965; see also Hubel *et al.*, 1977; Wiesel, 1982). Their studies focused primarily on the property of binocularity of cells in the primary visual cortex of cats, and later monkeys, and the destructive effects of reduced or absent visual input to one eye on binocular organization. On the basis of these early studies, Wiesel and Hubel suggested that amblyopia might result from a reduction in the number of neurons influenced by the deprived eye in primary visual cortex.

The demonstration of plasticity in the organization of ocular dominance spawned interest in the question of whether other properties of cortical cells could also be modified by early visual experience (see Movshon and van Sluyters, 1981; Movshon and Kiorpes, 1990). It became clear that other functional properties of visual cortical cells, for example orientation preference and direction selectivity, could be influenced by early visual experience. The important question, and the one that is of clinical interest, is: what properties of the visual system are affected by visual abnormalities that are associated with amblyopia in children? We know from clinical experience that anisometropia (a refractive difference between the eyes), strabismus (a misalignment of the two eyes) and unilateral cataract (an opacity in one eye), among other conditions, are associated with the development of amblyopia in children. When these same disorders appear in adults, they do not cause permanent visual deficits. Thus these disorders affect the developmental process. It is important, therefore, to understand the developmental mechanisms by which visual experience exerts its effects.

ANIMAL MODELS

To establish with certainty the causal nature of the relationship between abnormal visual input and the development of amblyopia, and to learn about the neural correlates of amblyopia, it is necessary to study an animal model. There are several important factors that motivate the study of an animal model in this case. First, except in areas where routine screening is conducted, clinicians rarely see infants before a visual disorder becomes obvious, and once the condition presents itself the clinician is typically obliged to begin a course of treatment. However, the clinical profile at the time of presentation may not reflect the original precipitating condition. Numerous studies have shown that abnormal early visual experience can induce strabismus or anisometropia (e.g. Quick *et al.*, 1989; Kiorpes and Wallman, 1995; Smith *et al.*, 1999). Thus it is in many cases difficult to establish the age of onset and the actual cause of the amblyopia, or indeed whether the amblyopia was the result or itself the cause of the child's condition (Almeder *et al.*, 1990; Kiorpes and Wallman, 1995; see also Tyschen, 1993). Second, because of the need for clinical intervention in the case of an infant or child, it is difficult to study the natural course of amblyopia development in humans. Knowledge of the natural course of amblyopia development would be of particular value for decisions about the necessity of treatment, and the likely outcome and timing of particular courses of treatment. Finally, it is impossible with currently available methods to study the neural basis of amblyopia in human infants and children. To truly understand the condition and effectively treat it, knowledge of the neural mechanisms involved in amblyopia development is essential.

Most animal studies on visual system development are conducted with cats or macaque monkeys as subjects. The macaque monkey visual system is the better model of the two. The early visual pathways in macaques have been shown to be structurally and functionally similar to those in humans. Visual acuity and contrast sensitivity, two basic descriptors of visual function, are similar in macaques and humans (DeValois *et al.*, 1974; Williams *et al.*, 1981; Kiorpes and Movshon, 1990). Moreover, the course of visual acuity development in human and macaque infants is essentially identical if human and monkey age are scaled appropriately: monkey age in weeks is approximately equivalent to human age in months (Teller, 1981, 1997; Boothe *et al.*, 1985; Kiorpes, 1992a; see Figure 1.1). The most important consideration for understanding amblyopia, though, is whether visual conditions that are associated with amblyopia in children also result in amblyopia in monkeys. We have shown that infant monkeys naturally develop strabismus, and do so with a frequency similar to that in humans (Kiorpes and Boothe, 1981; Kiorpes *et al.*, 1985). Amblyopia develops in monkeys in association with naturally occurring strabismus (Kiorpes, 1989); amblyopia also develops when a strabismus is created experimentally under controlled conditions early in life in an otherwise normal animal (von Noorden and Dowling, 1970; Kiorpes and Boothe, 1980; Harwerth *et al.*,

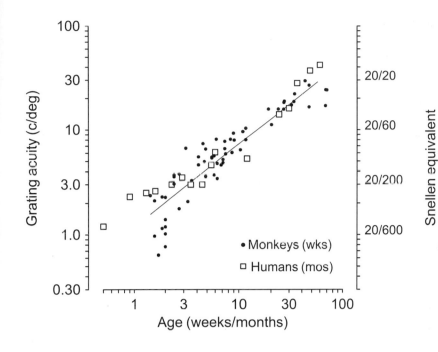

Figure 1.1 *Comparison of visual acuity development in human and macaque monkey infants. Grating acuity in c/deg is plotted as a function of age in weeks for the monkey infants (filled circles) and age in months for the human infants (open squares); Snellen equivalent acuity is shown on the right ordinate. When age is scaled in this way, it is clear that development follows a similar time course in these two primate species. Human data are from Mayer and Dobson (1982).*

1983; Kiorpes *et al.*, 1989). Similarly, anisometropia, natural or experimentally simulated, can cause the development of amblyopia in macaque monkeys (Smith *et al.*, 1985; Kiorpes *et al.*, 1987, 1993; Smith *et al.*, 1999).

Studies of experimentally induced anisometropia and strabismus in monkeys have shown unequivocally that the presence of unequal refractive error between the two eyes or misalignment of the visual axes during the early postnatal period is sufficient to cause the development of amblyopia. Reports of naturally occurring strabismus and anisometropia in monkeys confirms the close similarity between human and monkey visual systems. Furthermore, it has been demonstrated that naturally strabismic monkeys show visuomotor deficits that are similar to those identified in human congenital esotropes (Distler, 1996; Tyschen and Boothe, 1996). Abnormalities of smooth pursuit eye movements (Kiorpes *et al.*, 1996), binocularity, and stereopsis (Crawford *et al.*, 1983; Harwerth *et al.*, 1997) have been demonstrated in experimentally strabismic monkeys in addition to amblyopia. Collectively, these results strengthen the utility of the monkey model for understanding strabismus, anisometropia and amblyopia.

Cats are less desirable as a model species for amblyopia, primarily because the organization of their visual system is somewhat different from that of primates, and adult visual acuity is considerably poorer than that of humans and monkeys (see Kiorpes and Movshon, 1990). Also, the profile of visual acuity development is quite different from the primate pattern in that acuity improves rapidly over a short period of time following eye opening, and asymptotes by 10–12 weeks at adult levels (Mitchell *et al.*, 1976). However, visual abnormalities of the kind that lead to amblyopia in monkeys can result in reduced visual acuity in cats as well, although the deficits tend to be small and in many cases the cats become bilaterally amblyopic (von Grünau and Singer, 1980; Holopigian and Blake, 1983; Mitchell *et al.*, 1984; see also Mitchell, 1988).

It must be noted that many studies of the effects of monocular deprivation (by lid suture or occlusion) on visual system development have been conducted in cats and in monkeys. Behavioural studies have shown that residual visual function following monocular deprivation is typically extremely poor, if measurable at all (Harwerth *et al.*, 1983, 1989; see also Movshon and Kiorpes, 1990; Mitchell, 1991). Such dramatic visual deficits are rare in human amblyopia, therefore this paradigm is not especially useful for understanding amblyopia generally. However, monocular deprivation is a reasonable model for understanding the effects of very dense congenital cataracts on visual system development. Also, monocular deprivation and reverse deprivation studies have been important for establishing the effects of particular treatment regimens on recovery of visual system function (Blakemore *et al.*, 1978; Crawford *et al.*, 1989; Harwerth *et al.*, 1989; Mitchell, 1991). A related model that has been especially useful for studying treatment regimes following cataract surgery is unilateral aphakia. Boothe and colleagues have developed a primate model that very closely mimics the human condition of aphakic amblyopia, which develops following removal of the natural lens to correct unilateral congenital cataract (O'Dell *et al.*, 1989; Boothe *et al.*, 1996).

Critical period

As noted above, amblyopia is a disorder of development; the conditions associated with amblyopia in childhood do not result in permanent visual deficits when they appear in adults. Thus there is a critical period for amblyopia development. The extent of the critical period in humans is a matter of some debate, but it is commonly thought to include the first 8 years after birth (von Noorden, 1980). It is important to realize, though, that there are multiple aspects to the critical period (see Daw, 1995, 1998); the critical period is not necessarily synonymous with the period of visual development, and treatment efficacy is not equivalent throughout. Harwerth and colleagues (1986, 1989) have shown, using a deprivation model in monkeys, that different visual functions have different critical periods. For example, spatial vision can be compromised at a later age than spectral sensitivity, and the period of vulnerability of spatial vision extends beyond the period of normal development of spatial vision in macaques. Also, as noted below, we find improvements, as well as losses, in spatial vision of amblyopes beyond the period of normal visual development in macaques.

Daw (1998) points out that for visual acuity there are really three sub-periods, which are not mutually exclusive, that need to be considered: the period of normal visual development, the period within which amblyopia can develop, and the period within which amblyopia can be successfully treated.

For humans, most studies show that adult levels of visual acuity are reached between 3 and 5 years (Mayer and Dobson, 1982; Birch *et al.*, 1983; Teller, 1997), although improvements in contrast sensitivity and vernier acuity have been noted to continue beyond 5 years (Bradley and Freeman, 1982; Abramov *et al.*, 1984; Carkeet *et al.*, 1997). One recent retrospective study of amblyopia development found that children's susceptibility to amblyopia development declined by 6 years (Keech and Kutschke, 1995), but it has been reported that treatment for amblyopia can be at least partially effective into the teenage years (see Daw, 1998). To compare monkey and human critical periods we can use the age translation mentioned above, that monkey age in weeks is approximately equivalent to human age in months (Teller, 1981). In monkeys, the development of acuity and contrast sensitivity is complete by the end of the first postnatal year (Boothe *et al.*, 1988), which translates to 4.3 human years, and contrast sensitivity can be degraded by deprivation as late as 18 months (Harwerth *et al.*, 1986), which translates to 6 human years. No data are available on the upper limit for treatment of amblyopia in monkeys. However, it has been demonstrated, across conditions and species studied (including humans), that early intervention can reduce or completely reverse the effects of early abnormal visual experience, whereas later in the critical period treatment becomes less effective (e.g. Crawford and von Noorden, 1979; Crawford *et al.*, 1989; Birch *et al.*, 1990, 1998; Mitchell, 1991). The similarity in developmental profiles and critical periods strengthens the point that the macaque monkey is an excellent model for human visual development and for studying the vulnerability of the human visual system to abnormal visual experience.

Natural course of amblyopia development

The natural course of amblyopia development has been documented in strabismic monkeys (Kiorpes, 1989, 1992b; Kiorpes *et al.*, 1989). Naturally strabismic monkeys studied longitudinally showed normal acuity in each eye during the early postnatal weeks, but some time later, beyond 8–10 weeks, most developed amblyopia. A similar pattern was noted by Birch and Stager (1985) in a prospective study of human infantile esotropes. Of the six cases of early onset strabismus studied in monkeys, four cases developed amblyopia and two cases did not (one was an alternating esotrope and the other was an exotrope); two cases that initially developed amblyopia showed a reduction in the degree of amblyopia by 2–3 years of age (Kiorpes, 1989). One other case that was studied developed strabismus and anisometropia following bilateral congenital cataracts; this animal also became amblyopic. One particularly intriguing finding was that the naturally strabismic monkeys seemed to show a protracted developmental time course compared to normal animals. These monkeys continued to show improvement in acuity and contrast sensitivity through the second postnatal year, whereas normal monkeys reach adult levels on these measures by the end of the first postnatal year.

We found a similar pattern of development in longitudinal studies of experimentally strabismic monkeys (Kiorpes *et al.*, 1989; Kiorpes, 1992b). In

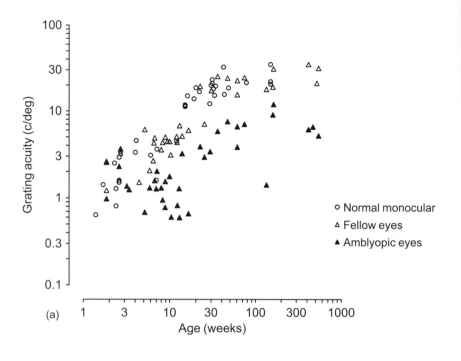

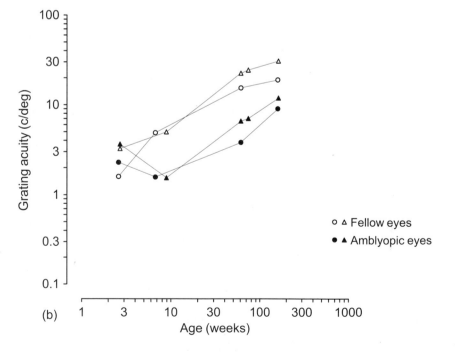

Figure 1.2 *Acuity development in strabismic monkeys. (a) Grating acuity is plotted as a function of age for amblyopic eyes (filled triangles) and fellow eyes (open triangles) of monkeys with experimentally induced esotropia. Control data (open circles) are from normal infants tested monocularly. (b) Longitudinal acuity development is shown for each eye of two monkeys with surgical esotropia induced at 3.5 weeks postnatal. Open symbols represent fellow eye data; filled symbols represent amblyopic eye data.*

these studies, esotropia was induced either by surgical alteration of the horizontal rectus muscles or by injection of *Oculinum* (C. *Botulinum A* neurotoxin) into the lateral rectus muscle at ages ranging from 1 to 15 weeks postnatal. On average, 67 per cent of experimentally strabismic monkeys developed amblyopia, defined as a factor of two or greater deficit in acuity for the deviated eye compared to the fellow eye. Age of onset was an important factor in determining which animals developed amblyopia. Amblyopia developed in 80 per cent of cases when esotropia was induced within the first 4 postnatal weeks, whereas 50 per cent developed amblyopia with later ages of onset. Fixation pattern was another important predictor of amblyopia: those monkeys that alternated fixation were less likely to develop amblyopia than those that adopted a unilateral fixation pattern. The longitudinal acuity data show that the time course of acuity development for the deviated eyes lagged behind that for the fellow eyes (see Figure 1.2); in some cases acuity in the deviated eye actually declined initially, whereas in other cases there was a delay in development followed by a resumption of the developmental time course thereafter. This pattern of delayed or slowed development was also found using other measures of visual function, such as contrast sensitivity and vernier acuity (Kiorpes, 1992b; Kiorpes, 1996).

Characteristics of amblyopia in the monkey

Although amblyopia is most commonly identified clinically as a deficit in acuity, the full contrast sensitivity function is a more complete descriptor of visual function. The contrast sensitivity function provides information about visual sensitivity at all spatial scales, from coarse to fine, whereas acuity provides a measure only of fine resolution. Normal adult monkeys (and humans) show similar contrast sensitivity functions for the right and left eyes and enhanced contrast sensitivity under binocular viewing conditions (Figure 1.3a). Amblyopes show deficits in contrast sensitivity at the high spatial frequencies (fine spatial scale), as would be expected given the acuity deficit, but they also typically show losses for mid-range spatial frequencies and occasionally for low spatial frequencies as well (Figure 1.3b). The binocular enhancement seen in normal observers is typically absent in amblyopic observers (Harwerth and Levi, 1983); our monkey amblyopes also failed to show binocular summation for contrast sensitivity. Similar results have been reported by other labs (Harwerth *et al.*, 1983; Smith *et al.*, 1985). The deficits in contrast sensitivity in amblyopic monkeys are reminiscent of contrast sensitivity profiles in infants. Boothe *et al.* (1988) showed that infant monkeys have low sensitivity to contrast over the range of spatial scales to which they are sensitive, and that the spatial scale of the infant visual system is shifted to a much lower range than that of adults (Figure 1.3c). As development proceeds, the contrast sensitivity function shifts upward and to the right, to higher spatial scales and higher contrast sensitivity. If we directly compare normal infant and amblyopic adult contrast sensitivity functions, we find that the amblyopic functions resemble data from younger normal monkeys (Kiorpes, 1996). Hence, in terms of this basic descriptor of visual function,

Figure 1.3 *Contrast sensitivity functions for normal and amblyopic monkeys. Contrast sensitivity is plotted as a function of spatial frequency; high spatial frequencies represent fine spatial scales. (a) Contrast sensitivity for a normal adult monkey. Open and filled circles and solid curves represent left and right eye data; open triangles and broken curve represent binocular data. (b) Contrast sensitivity for a strabismic amblyopic monkey. Open and filled circles represent fellow and amblyopic eye data, respectively; open triangles represent data collected with binocular viewing. Note that binocular viewing does not improve sensitivity for the amblyopic monkey, suggesting a lack of binocular summation. (c) Contrast sensitivity for a normal monkey at two ages: 5 weeks (filled circles) and 20 weeks (open circles). The contrast sensitivity function shifts up to higher sensitivity and over to finer spatial scales with development.*

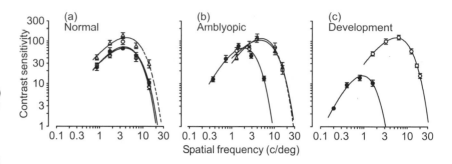

amblyopia does not represent a completely disordered or abnormal state of visual function. Rather, amblyopia can be characterized as an incompletely developed visual system.

Our studies of the development of vernier acuity led us to a similar conclusion. Studies of human amblyopes had shown that they were particularly impaired on spatial localization tasks in comparison to their deficits in grating and Snellen acuity. Strabismic amblyopes in particular were substantially more impaired on localization tasks compared to anisometropic amblyopes (e.g. Levi and Klein, 1982, 1985; Hess *et al.*, 1990). To investigate whether the development of vernier and grating acuity proceed along the same time course, and to see whether the development of these functions is similarly disrupted in amblyopia, we studied the development of vernier acuity and grating acuity longitudinally in normal animals, and also in animals who had experimentally-induced strabismus (Kiorpes, 1992a, 1992b). We found that vernier acuity in normal infants is relatively less mature than grating acuity, and develops to a greater extent during the first postnatal year. Therefore, the two functions do not show the same developmental profile, although adult levels are approached at similar ages. A recent study in human infants has shown the same developmental relationship between vernier acuity and grating acuity that we found for monkeys (Skoczenski and Norcia, 1999; see also Levi and Carkeet, 1993).

Strabismus disrupted vernier acuity development as well as grating acuity development. The disruption of vernier acuity development was similar to that described above for the development of grating acuity and contrast sensitivity: vernier acuity development in amblyopic eyes lagged behind the fellow eyes and proceeded more slowly. When these monkeys were tested as adults, the deficit in vernier acuity was larger than the deficit in grating acuity, which is consistent with what has been reported in humans. However, this relatively larger vernier acuity loss may be the result of the different developmental profiles we identified for vernier and grating acuity. Since vernier acuity in normal infants is relatively less mature than grating acuity and develops to a greater extent, and since the developmental time course is slower for amblyopes, the relatively greater impairment of vernier acuity over grating acuity may simply be a reflection of a less mature visual system at the end of the critical period rather than a peculiar deficit in positional acuity (Kiorpes, 1992b).

While our studies showed the expected superordinate loss in positional acuity, we did not find a clear distinction between anisometropic and strabismic amblyopes in the relationship between vernier acuity and grating acuity impairment that has been reported in human psychophysical studies (Levi and Klein, 1985; see also Chapter 2). We induced anisometropic amblyopia by rearing macaques with unilateral defocus; defocus was imposed with extended-wear contact lenses. While we did not study the development of anisometropic amblyopia longitudinally, we measured vernier acuity as well as other visual functions after the end of the rearing period, at about 1 year of age (Kiorpes *et al.*, 1993). Like our strabismic amblyopes, the anisometropic amblyopes showed a relatively larger deficit in vernier acuity, although the effect was on balance somewhat smaller for the anisometropes than for the strabismics. To see if this was a fundamental species difference or not, we compared our monkey data directly with data from a population of human amblyopes (Kiorpes and Movshon, 1996). We used data from the Cooperative Amblyopia Classification Study (McKee *et al.*, 1992; Movshon *et al.*, 1996), which included measurements of vernier and grating acuity in a large group of amblyopes with known clinical histories. As shown in Figure 1.4, the amblyopic monkeys fell well within the range of the data from human amblyopes. Interestingly, like our monkeys, this large group of human amblyopes does not show a clear distinction between anisometropic and

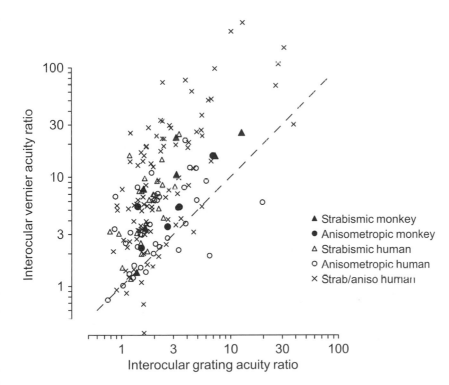

Figure 1.4 *Comparison between the deficit in vernier acuity and the deficit in grating acuity for human and monkey amblyopes. The extent of the amblyopic deficit on each measure is presented as an interocular ratio: fellow eye acuity/amblyopic eye acuity. The dashed line represents a slope of 1. If the data clustered along the line, the deficits on each measure would be equal. However, since the data are largely scattered above the line, the deficits in vernier acuity are larger than those in grating acuity. Circles represent anisometropic amblyopes and triangles represent strabismic amblyopes; filled symbols represent monkey subjects and open symbols represent human subjects. The crosses are data from human combined strabismic-anisometropes. Human data are from McKee* et al., *1992; Movshon* et al., *1996; see also Kiorpes and Movshon, 1996.*

▲ Strabismic monkey
● Anisometropic monkey
△ Strabismic human
○ Anisometropic human
× Strab/aniso human

strabismic observers in the relative extent of the deficit in vernier acuity. Mixed strabismic–anisometropic observers tend to show the most extreme deficits in vernier acuity. We have not explicitly modelled this condition, although some of our experimentally strabismic, amblyopic monkeys later developed anisometropia, and some experimentally anisometropic monkeys later developed a natural anisometropia or strabismus (Kiorpes and Wallman, 1995; Kiorpes *et al.*, 1999).

These psychophysical studies of monkeys with strabismic and anisometropic amblyopia show many of the characteristics that are considered basic to human amblyopia. In addition to the deficits in acuity, contrast sensitivity and spatial localization already described, we have identified deficits in spatial phase discrimination (Kiper, 1994), suprathreshold contrast sensitivity (Kiper and Kiorpes, 1994), motion sensitivity (Tang *et al.*, 1998) and contour integration (Kozma *et al.*, 2000). Some of these deficits can be explained on the basis of the primary loss of contrast sensitivity, as is true for many human amblyopes. Furthermore, a psychophysical study designed to determine whether the primary site of the contrast sensitivity deficit in amblyopia is early in the visual pathways or perhaps in the central pathways (cortical) suggested that the loss is predominantly central (Kiorpes *et al.*, 1999). Physiological studies in some of the same animals confirmed that deficits can be found in the visual cortex that reflect, at least qualitatively, the behavioural losses (Kiorpes *et al.*, 1998).

Neural correlates of amblyopia

As noted at the beginning of this chapter, the early studies of Hubel and Wiesel and others suggested that the primary neural correlate of amblyopia was a dramatic reduction in the number of neurons in the primary visual cortex (V1) that could be influenced by the deprived eye. However, looking back over several decades of work, we find that a breakdown of binocular function is a ubiquitous result in strabismus, anisometropia and deprivation, but a dramatic deficit in amblyopic eye activity in V1 is not a consistent correlate of amblyopia. The breakdown of binocular function is characterized by a dearth of neurons that can be influenced relatively equally by each eye. Interestingly, recent studies have shown that although the classical test of ocular dominance suggests a lack of binocular function, there can be residual binocular interactions (Sengpiel and Blakemore, 1996; Smith *et al.*, 1997). These studies show that there are indeed deficient excitatory interactions, but that inhibitory, suppressive interactions persist following anisometropic (lens-rearing) and strabismic (prism-rearing or surgical strabismus) early rearing. The relationship between these residual binocular interactions and the presence of amblyopia is not clear, though. The anisometropic animals studied by Smith and colleagues all showed deficits in contrast sensitivity at high spatial frequencies, but the prism-reared animals had comparatively small deficits or no deficits. Nevertheless, both groups showed measurable binocular interactions at the single-cell level.

The appearance of a shift of cortical ocular dominance away from the amblyopic eye seems to be different for strabismic amblyopia and for blur or deprivation-induced amblyopia. The majority of studies of anisometropic or deprivation-induced amblyopia, in which the presence of amblyopia was behaviourally verified, show a reduction in the number of neurons driven by the amblyopic eye (Baker et al., 1974; Movshon et al., 1987; Kiorpes et al., 1998; but see also Smith et al., 1997). This is not a consistent finding in strabismic amblyopia. Some studies find balanced influence from the two eyes in strabismic amblyopes with mild to moderate amblyopia (see Figure 1.5b; Smith et al., 1997; Kiorpes et al., 1998), whereas others report a shift away from the amblyopic eye even in relatively mild amblyopia (Wiesel, 1982). However, deep strabismic amblyopia does tend to be associated with a reduction of influence by the deviated eye (Baker et al., 1974; Crawford and von Noorden, 1979; Kiorpes et al., 1998). On balance, a shift of cortical influence away from the amblyopic eye seems to be associated with relatively severe amblyopia, deprivation, or blur-rearing, but is not reliably associated with strabismus or mild to moderate amblyopia. Thus, it is important to look beyond the idea of a simple imbalance in cortical influence as the basis of amblyopia.

Since amblyopia is predominantly a disorder of spatial vision, it is important to evaluate the spatial properties of neurons in the visual pathways. Only a few studies have made quantitative assessments of spatial properties of neurons in amblyopic animals. Movshon and co-workers (1987) studied spatial tuning properties of V1 neurons in monkeys raised with chronic unilateral defocus from daily instillation of atropine in one eye; behavioural testing of contrast sensitivity showed that these animals developed amblyopia (Kiorpes et al., 1987). Consistent with the behavioural deficits in contrast sensitivity, neurons driven by the treated eyes were found to have a reduction in overall contrast sensitivity, preferred spatial frequency and spatial resolution compared with neurons driven by the untreated eyes. These deficits were not reflected in the physiological properties of neurons earlier in the visual pathways, in the LGN (see also Blakemore and Vital-Durand, 1986). Eggers and Blakemore (1978) reported similar results in cats reared with monocular optical defocus. They found a reduction in contrast sensitivity and spatial resolution of V1 neurons driven by the treated eye; however, they did not test their animals behaviourally to verify the presence of amblyopia.

Kiorpes and co-workers (1998) studied spatial tuning properties of V1 neurons in animals that were behaviourally verified to be strabismic or anisometropic amblyopes. Strabismus was induced surgically (Kiorpes et al., 1989); anisometropia was simulated during rearing with defocusing contact lenses (Kiorpes et al., 1993). Full contrast sensitivity functions were measured to document the presence of amblyopia (see Figure 1.5a). This study showed a clear correlation between the behavioural deficits in spatial vision and reduced spatial frequency sensitivity in V1 neurons. For animals with moderate to severe amblyopia, the range of preferred spatial frequency and spatial resolution for amblyopic eye neurons was shifted to lower spatial scale with respect to those for fellow eye neurons (Figure 1.5c). A similar reduction

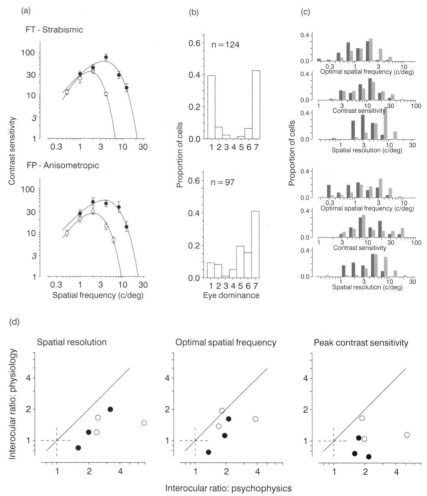

Figure 1.5 *Comparison of behavioural and physiological correlates of amblyopia. (a) Contrast sensitivity functions for one strabismic (top) and one anisometropic (bottom) amblyopic monkey (filled symbols represent fellow eye data; open symbols represent amblyopic eye data). Note that the depth of amblyopia is similar for each case. (b) Ocular dominance histograms for the monkeys in (a). These histograms show the proportion of cells in primary visual cortex that could be influenced by either eye. The strabismic monkey (top) showed equal representation of the fellow (dominance category 7) and amblyopic (dominance category 1) eye, while the anisometropic monkey showed a skewed distribution: many fewer cells could be driven by the amblyopic eye than the fellow eye. For both monkeys, relatively few cells were binocular (dominance categories 2–6). (c) Distributions of optimal (preferred) spatial frequency, contrast sensitivity, and spatial resolution for neurons tested through the amblyopic (dark bars) and fellow (light bars) eye of the same two monkeys. The distributions of optimal frequency and spatial resolution for amblyopic eye neurons of each monkey were significantly lower than the distributions for fellow eye neurons. The distributions for contrast sensitivity were not significantly different for amblyopic and fellow eye neurons in these cases. (d) Quantitative comparison of the extent of the behavioural and physiological deficits in anisometropic and strabismic amblyopes. For each measure, the interocular ratios for physiologically assessed neural sensitivity are plotted against those for behavioural sensitivity. Open and filled circles represent data from anisometropic and strabismic animals, respectively. If the behavioural and physiological deficits were commensurate, the data would cluster along the diagonal drawn through each plot; the data fall largely below the diagonals indicating a larger behavioural than physiological deficit. Data are from Kiorpes et al., 1998.*

in neuronal acuity has been reported in strabismic cats with behaviourally documented acuity losses (Chino *et al.*, 1983; Crewther and Crewther, 1990). The shift to lower preferred spatial frequency and resolution mimics that seen behaviourally, with the shift of the contrast sensitivity function to a lower spatial scale for the amblyopic eye. As Figure 1.5d shows, there was a reliable relationship between the extent of the behavioural deficit and the extent of the physiological one, although the physiological shift was typically smaller than the behavioural deficit. Consistent with the finding that the physiological deficits were smaller than the behavioural deficits, the mildest amblyopes showed no reliable difference between the amblyopic and fellow eye distributions. Curiously, unlike the earlier study (Movshon *et al.*, 1987), there was no consistent effect on neuronal contrast sensitivity even in the deepest amblyopes. Overall, the range of contrast sensitivities for amblyopic eye neurons was similar to that for fellow eye neurons. This latter result, and the finding that the spatial deficit apparent in the neuronal population is smaller than the behavioural deficit, led us to conclude that neural correlates of amblyopia can be seen at the level of single neurons in V1, but that it is likely that these deficits are amplified and probably compounded at subsequent levels of processing either within or beyond V1.

The extraordinary deficit in spatial localization ability in amblyopia, which is particularly apparent in strabismic and mixed amblyopes, cannot easily be explained on the basis of this physiological deficit in spatial frequency sensitivity. Several psychophysical theories have been proposed to explain the spatial localization deficit, most notably that there is a topographical jitter or disarray in the amblyopic eye neurons' receptive fields, or that there is under-sampling of the amblyopic visual world at fine spatial scales (see, for example, Hess *et al.*, 1999; Kiorpes and McKee, 1999; Levi *et al.*, 1999; and Chapter 2). Our finding that the range of spatial scale sensitivity of amblyopic eye neurons is lower than for fellow eye neurons could provide a substrate for under-sampling at fine spatial scales. However, while receptive fields for amblyopic eye neurons did not appear to be disordered with respect to nearby fellow eye neurons, it would be difficult to capture disarray at the single unit level without finer sampling. The question of topographic disarray may be better addressed at a higher, perhaps extrastriate, level of the visual system where receptive fields integrate over larger areas of visual space.

Finally, it is informative to compare the physiological properties of amblyopic neurons to those of normal infants. Physiological studies of foveal V1 neurons in 1–4-week-old monkeys show that, on average, preferred spatial frequency is two to three times lower than that found in adult monkeys, while orientation and direction selectivity are essentially adult-like in newborns (Movshon *et al.*, 1999, 2000; see also Chino *et al.*, 1997). Spatial resolution of infant V1 neurons is about a factor of 5 lower than in adults (Blakemore, 1990; Chino *et al.*, 1997). In our amblyopes, spatial resolution and preferred spatial frequency was a factor of 1.5–2 lower for neurons driven by amblyopic eyes compared to neurons driven by the fellow eyes, while orientation and direction selectivity were normal in all cases. These results suggest that receptive field properties that are immature in infants are affected by the abnormal visual input that leads to amblyopia; these properties develop from newborn levels, but do so more slowly, or perhaps incompletely, in the presence of abnormal visual input. Thus, as indicated by our longitudinal behavioural studies of strabismic and anisometropic monkeys, a slowed developmental time course may leave the visual system in an immature state at the end of the critical period.

CONCLUSION

This chapter has attempted to convey the utility of the primate model for amblyopia, describe the relationship between strabismic and anisometropic amblyopia in monkeys (both experimentally induced and naturally occurring) and that which has been characterized in humans, and provide some insight into the developmental mechanisms that may underlie amblyopia. These studies have shown that amblyopia is a disorder of the developmental time course, and the slowed development is reflected initially in the spatial properties of V1 neurons. Numerous animal studies have been directed at the molecular mechanisms that control the period of visual plasticity and the progress of development (see Daw, 1995). Progress in this area may allow us to understand more completely the mechanisms of plasticity, and perhaps eventually allow us to extend the critical period, to more effectively treat amblyopia in children.

REFERENCES

Abramov, I., Hainline, L., Turkel, J. *et al.* (1984). Rocket-ship psychophysics: assessing visual functioning in young children. *Inv. Ophthalmol. Vis. Sci.*, **25**, 1307–15.

Almeder, L. M., Peck, L. B. and Howland, H. C. (1990). Prevalence of anisometropia in volunteer laboratory and school screening populations. *Inv. Ophthalmol. Vis. Sci.*, **31**, 2448–55.

Baker, F. H., Grigg, P. and von Noorden, G. (1974). Effects of visual deprivation and strabismus on the response of neurons in the visual cortex of the monkey, including studies of striate and prestriate cortex in the normal animal. *Brain Res.*, **66**, 185–208.

Birch, E. E and Stager, D. R. (1985). Monocular acuity and stereopsis in infantile esotropia. *Inv. Ophthalmol. Vis. Sci.*, **26**, 1624–30.

Birch, E. E, Gwiazda, J. A., Bauer, J. A. *et al.* (1983). Visual acuity and its meridional variations in children aged 7–60 months. *Vision Res.*, **23**, 1019–24.

Birch, E. E., Stager, D. R., Berry, P. and Everett, M. E. (1990). Prospective assessment of acuity and stereopsis in amblyopic infantile esotropes following early surgery. *Inv. Ophthalmol. Vis. Sci.*, **31**, 758–65.

Birch, E. E., Stager, D., Leffler, J. and Weakley, D. (1998). Early treatment of congenital unilateral cataract minimizes unequal competition. *Inv. Ophthalmol. Vis. Sci.,* **39**, 1560–66.

Blakemore, C. (1990). Maturation of mechanisms for efficient spatial vision. In: *Vision: Coding and Efficiency* (C. Blakemore, ed.), pp. 254–66. Cambridge University Press.

Blakemore, C. and Vital-Durand, F. (1986). Effects of visual deprivation on the development of the monkey's lateral geniculate nucleus. *J. Physiol.*, **380**, 493–511.

Blakemore, C., Garey, L. J. and Vital-Durand, F. (1978). The physiological effects of monocular deprivation and their reversal in the monkey's visual cortex. *J. Physiol.*, **283**, 223–62.

Boothe, R. G., Dobson, V. and Teller, D. Y. (1985). Postnatal development of vision in human and non-human primates. *Ann. Rev. Neurosci.*, **8**, 495–545.

Boothe, R. G, Kiorpes, L., Williams, R. A. and Teller, D. Y. (1988). Operant measurements of contrast sensitivity in infant macaque monkeys during normal development. *Vision Res.*, **28**, 387–96.

Boothe, R. G., Louden, T. M. and Lambert, S. R. (1996). Acuity and contrast sensitivity in monkeys after neonatal intraocular lens implantation with and without part time occlusion of the fellow eye. *Inv. Ophthalmol. Vis. Sci.*, **37**, 1520–31.

Bradley, A. and Freeman, R. D. (1982). Contrast sensitivity in children. *Vision Res.*, **22**, 953–9.

Carkeet, A., Levi, D. M. and Manny, R. E. (1997). Development of vernier acuity in childhood. *Optom. Vis. Sci.*, **74**, 741–50.

Chino, Y. M., Shansky, M. S., Jankowski, W. L. and Banser, F. A. (1983). Effects of rearing kittens with convergent strabismus on development of receptive-field properties in striate cortex neurons. *J. Neurophysiol.*, **50**, 265–86.

Chino, Y. M., Smith, E. L., Hatta, S. and Cheng. H. (1997). Postnatal development of binocular disparity in neurons of the primate visual cortex. *J. Neurosci.*, **17**, 296–307.

Crawford, M. L. J. and von Noorden, G. K. (1979). The effects of short-term experimental strabismus on the visual system in *Macaca mulatta*. *Inv. Ophthalmol. Vis. Sci.*, **18**, 496 505.

Crawford, M. L. J., von Noorden, G. K. and Meharg, L. S. *et al.* (1983). Binocular neurons and binocular function in monkeys and children. *Inv. Ophthalmol. Vis. Sci.*, **24**, 491–5.

Crawford, M. L. J., de Faber, J.-T. and Harwerth, R. S. *et al.* (1989). The effects of reverse monocular deprivation in monkeys. II. Electrophysiological and anatomical studies. *Exp. Brain Res.*, **74**, 338–47.

Crewther, D. P. and Crewther, S. G. (1990). Neural site of strabismic amblyopia in cats: spatial frequency deficit in primary cortical neurons. *Exp. Brain Res.*, **79**, 615–22.

Daw, N. W. (1995). *Visual Development*. Plenum.

Daw, N. W. (1998). Critical periods and amblyopia. *Arch. Ophthalmol.*, **116**, 502–5.

De Valois, R. L., Morgan, H. and Snodderly, D. M. (1974). Psychophysical studies of monkey vision – III. Spatial luminance contrast sensitivity tests of macaque and human observers. *Vision Res.*, **14**, 75–81.

Distler, C. (1996). Neuronal basis of optokinetic reflex pathology in naturally strabismic monkeys. *Strabismus*, **4**, 111–26.

Eggers, H. M. and Blakemore, C. (1978). Physiological basis of anisometropic amblyopia. *Science*, **201**, 264–7.

Harwerth, R. S. and Levi, D. M. (1983). Psychophysical studies on the binocular processes of amblyopes. *Am. J. Optom. Physiol. Optics*, **60**, 454–63.

Harwerth, R. S., Smith, E. L., Boltz, R. L. *et al.* (1983). Behavioral studies on the effect of abnormal early visual experience: Spatial modulation sensitivity. *Vision Res.*, **23**, 1501–10.

Harwerth, R. S., Smith, E. L., Duncan, G. C. *et al.* (1986). Multiple sensitive periods in the development of the primate visual system. *Science*, **232**, 235–8.

Harwerth, R. S., Smith, E. L., Crawford, M. L. J. and von Noorden, G. K. (1989). The effects of reverse monocular deprivation in monkeys. I. Psychophysical experiments. *Exp. Brain Res.*, **74**, 327–37.

Harwerth, R. S., Smith, E. L., Crawford, M. L. J. and von Noorden, G. K. (1997). Stereopsis and disparity vergence in monkeys with subnormal binocular vision. *Vision Res.*, **37**, 483–93.

Hess, R. F., Field, D. J. and Watt, R. J. (1990). The puzzle of amblyopia. In: *Vision: Coding and Efficiency* (C. Blakemore, ed.), pp. 267–80. Cambridge University Press.

Hess, R. F., Wang, Y.-Z., Demanins, R. *et al.* (1999). A deficit in strabismic amblyopia for global shape detection. *Vision Res.*, **39**, 901–14.

Holopigian, K. and Blake, R. (1983). Spatial vision in strabismic cats. *J. Neurophysiol.*, **50**, 287–96.

Hubel, D. H., Wiesel, T. N. and LeVay, S. (1977). Plasticity of ocular dominance columns in monkey striate cortex. *Philosophical Trans. R. Soc. Lond. Series B*, **278**, 377–409.

Keech, R. V. and Kutschke, P. J. (1995). Upper age limit for the development of amblyopia. *J. Ped. Ophthalmol. Strab.*, **32**, 89–93.

Kiorpes, L. (1989). The development of spatial resolution and contrast sensitivity in naturally strabismic monkeys. *Clin. Vision Sci.*, **4**, 279–93.

Kiorpes, L. (1992a). Development of vernier acuity and grating acuity in normally reared monkeys. *Vis. Neurosci.*, **9**, 243–51.

Kiorpes, L. (1992b). Effect of strabismus on the development of vernier acuity and grating acuity in monkeys. *Vis. Neurosci.*, **9**, 253–9.

Kiorpes, L. (1996). Development of contrast sensitivity in normal and amblyopic monkeys. In: *Infant Vision* (F. Vital-Durand, J. Atkinson and O. J. Braddick, eds), pp. 2–15. Oxford University Press.

Kiorpes, L. and Boothe, R. G. (1980). The time course for the development of strabismic amblyopia in infant monkeys. *Inv. Ophthalmol. Vis. Sci.*, **19**, 841–5.

Kiorpes, L. and Boothe, R. G. (1981). Naturally occurring strabismus in monkeys. *Inv. Ophthalmol. Vis. Sci.*, **20**, 257–63.

Kiorpes, L. and McKee, S. P. (1999). Neural mechanisms underlying amblyopia. *Curr. Opin. Neurobiol.*, **9**, 480–86.

Kiorpes, L. and Movshon, J. A. (1990). Behavioral analysis of visual development. In: *Development of Sensory Systems in Mammals* (J. R. Coleman, ed.), pp. 125–54. Wiley.

Kiorpes, L. and Movshon, J. A. (1996). Amblyopia: a developmental disorder of the central visual pathways. *Cold Spring Harbor Symposium on Quantitative Biology*, **LXI**, 39–48.

Kiorpes, L. and Wallman, J. (1995). Does experimentally-induced amblyopia cause hyperopia in monkeys? *Vision Res.*, **35**, 1289–97.

Kiorpes, L., Boothe, R. G., Carlson, M. R. and Alfi, D. A. (1985). Frequency of naturally occurring strabismus in monkeys. *J. Ped. Ophthalmol. Strab.*, **22**, 60–64.

Kiorpes, L., Boothe, R. G., Hendrickson, A. E. *et al.* (1987). Effects of early unilateral blur on the macaque's visual system. I. Behavioral observations. *J. Neurosci.*, **7**, 1318–26.

Kiorpes, L., Carlson, M. R. and Alfi, D. (1989). Development of visual acuity in experimentally strabismic monkeys. *Clin. Vision Sci.*, **4**, 95–106.

Kiorpes, L., Kiper, D. C. and Movshon, J. A. (1993). Contrast sensitivity and vernier acuity in amblyopic monkeys. *Vision Res.*, **33**, 2301–11.

Kiorpes, L., Walton, P. J., O'Keefe, L. P. *et al.* (1996). Effects of early-onset artificial strabismus on pursuit eye movements and on neuronal responses in area MT of macaque monkeys. *J. Neurosci.*, **16**, 6537–53.

Kiorpes, L., Kiper, D. C., O'Keefe, L. P. *et al.* (1998). Neuronal correlates of amblyopia in the visual cortex of macaque monkeys with experimental strabismus and anisometropia. *J. Neurosci.*, **18**, 6411–24.

Kiorpes, L., Tang, C. and Movshon, J. A. (1999). Factors limiting contrast sensitivity in experimentally amblyopic macaque monkeys. *Vision Res.*, **39**, 4152–60.

Kiper, D. C. (1994). Spatial phase discrimination in monkeys with experimental strabismus. *Vision Res.*, **34**, 437–47.

Kiper, D. C. and Kiorpes, L. (1994). Suprathreshold contrast sensitivity in experimentally strabismic monkeys. *Vision Res.*, **34**, 1575–83.

Kozma, P., Kiorpes, L. and Movshon, J. A. (2000). Contour intergration in amblyopic monkeys. *Inv. Ophthalmol. Vis. Sci.*, **41**, S703.

Levi, D. M. and Carkeet, A. (1993). Amblyopia: a consequence of abnormal visual development. In: *Early Visual Development: Normal and Abnormal* (K. Simons, ed.), pp. 391–408. Oxford University Press.

Levi, D. M. and Klein, S. A. (1982). Hyperacuity and amblyopia. *Nature (Lond.)*, **298**, 268–70.

Levi, D. M. and Klein, S. A. (1985). Vernier acuity, crowding, and amblyopia. *Vision Res.*, **25**, 979–91.

Levi, D. M., Klein, S. A. and Sharma, V. (1999). Position jitter and undersampling in pattern perception. *Vision Res.*, **39**, 445–65.

Mayer, D. L. and Dobson, V. (1982). Visual acuity development in infants and young children as assessed by operant preferential looking. *Vision Res.*, **22**, 1141–51.

McKee, S. P., Schor, C. M., Steinman, S. B. *et al.* (1992). The classification of amblyopia on the basis of visual and oculomotor performance. *Trans. Am. Ophthalmol. Soc.*, **90**, 123–48.

Mitchell, D. E. (1988). Animal models of human strabismic amblyopia: some observations concerning the interpretation of the effects of surgically and optically induced strabismus in cats and monkeys. In: *Advances in Neural and Behavioral Development*, Vol. 3 (P. G. Shinkman, ed.), pp. 209–69. Ablex.

Mitchell, D. E. (1991). The long-term effectiveness of different regimens of occlusion on recovery from early monocular deprivation in kittens. *Philosophical Trans. R. Soc. Lond. Series B*, **333**, 51–79.

Mitchell, D. E., Giffin, F., Wilkinson, F. *et al*. (1976). Visual resolution in young kittens. *Vision Res.*, **16**, 363–6.

Mitchell, D. E., Ruck, M., Kaye, M. G. and Kirby, S. (1984). Immediate and long-term effects on visual acuity of surgically induced strabismus in kittens. *Exp. Brain Res.*, **55**, 420–30.

Movshon, J. A. and Kiorpes, L. (1990). The role of experience in visual development. In: *Development of Sensory Systems in Mammals* (J. R. Coleman, ed.), pp. 155–202. Wiley.

Movshon, J. A. and van Sluyters, R. C. (1981). Visual neural development. *Ann. Rev. Psychol.*, **32**, 477–522.

Movshon, J. A., Eggers, H. M., Gizzi, M. S. *et al*. (1987). Effects of early unilateral blur on the macaque's visual system: III. Physiological observations. *J. Neurosci.*, **7**, 1340–51.

Movshon, J. A., McKee, S. P. and Levi, D. M. (1996). Visual acuity in a large population of normal, strabismic, and anisometropic observers. *Inv. Ophthalmol. Vis. Sci.*, **37**, S670.

Movshon, J. A., Kiorpes, L., Cavanaugh, J. R. and Hawken, M. J. (1999). Receptive field properties and surround interactions in V1 neurons in infant macaque monkeys. *Neurosci. Abstracts*, **25**, 1048.

Movshon, J. A., Kiorpes, L., Cavanaugh, J. R. and Hawken, M. J. (2000). Developmental reorganization of receptive field surrounds in V1 neurons in macaque monkeys. *Inv. Ophthalmol. Vis. Sci.*, **41**, S333.

O'Dell, C. D., Gammon, J. A., Fernandes, A. *et al*. (1989). Development of acuity in a primate model of human infantile unilateral aphakia. *Inv. Ophthalmol. Vis. Sci.*, **30**, 2068–74.

Quick, M. W., Tigges, M., Gammon, J. A. and Boothe, R. G. (1989). Early abnormal visual experience induces strabismus in infant monkeys. *Inv. Ophthalmol. Vis. Sci.*, **30**, 1012–17.

Sengpiel, F. and Blakemore, C. (1996). The neural basis of suppression and amblyopia in strabismus. *Eye*, **10**, 250–58.

Skoczenski, A. M. and Norcia, A. M. (1999). Development of VEP vernier acuity and grating acuity in human infants. *Inv. Ophthalmol. Vis. Sci.*, **40**, 2411–17.

Smith, E. L., Harwerth, R. S. and Crawford, M. L. J. (1985). Spatial contrast sensitivity deficits in monkeys produced by optically induced anisometropia. *Inv. Ophthalmol. Vis. Sci.*, **26**, 330–42.

Smith, E. L., Chino, Y. M., Ni, J. *et al*. (1997). Residual binocular interactions in the striate cortex of monkeys reared with abnormal binocular vision. *J. Neurophysiol.*, **78**, 1353–62.

Smith, E. L., Hung, L.-F. and Harwerth, R. S. (1999). Developmental visual system anomalies and the limits of emmetropization. *Ophthal. Physiol. Optics*, **19**, 90–102.

Tang, C., Kiorpes, L. and Movshon, J. A. (1998). Motion detection in amblyopic macaque monkeys. *Inv. Ophthalmol. Vis. Sci.*, **39**, S330.

Teller, D. Y. (1981). The development of visual acuity in human and monkey infants. *Trends Neurosci.*, **4**, 21–4.

Teller, D. Y. (1997). First glances: the vision of infants. *Inv. Ophthalmol. Vis. Sci.*, **38**, 2183–203.

Tychsen, L. (1993). Motion sensitivity and the origins of infantile strabismus. In: *Early Visual Development: Normal and Abnormal* (K. Simons, ed.), pp. 364–90. Oxford University Press.

Tychsen, L. and Boothe, R. G. (1996). Latent fixation nystagmus and nasotemporal asymmetries of motion visually evoked potentials in naturally strabismic primate. *J. Ped. Ophthalmol. Strab.*, **33**, 148–52.

von Grünau, M. W. and Singer, W. (1980). Functional amblyopia in kittens with unilateral exotropia. II. Correspondence between behavioural and electrophysiological assessment. *Exp. Brain Res.*, **40**, 305–10.

von Noorden, G. K. (1980). *Burian – Von Noorden's Binocular Vision and Ocular Motility*. C. V. Mosby.

von Noorden, G. K. and Dowling, J. E. (1970). Experimental amblyopia in monkeys. II. Behavioral studies of strabismic amblyopia. *Arch. Ophthalmol.*, **84,** 215–20.

Wiesel, T. N. (1982). Postnatal development of the visual cortex and the influence of environment. *Nature (Lond.)*, **299,** 583–91.

Wiesel, T. N. and Hubel, D. H. (1963). Single-cell responses in striate cortex of kittens deprived of vision in one eye. *J. Neurophysiol.*, **26,** 1003–17.

Wiesel, T. N. and Hubel, D. H. (1965). Comparison of the effects of unilateral and bilateral eye closure on cortical unit responses in kittens. *J. Neurophysiol.*, **28,** 1029–40.

Williams, R. A., Boothe, R. G., Kiorpes, L. and Teller, D. Y. (1981). Oblique effects in normally reared monkeys (*Macaca nemestrina*): meridional variations in contrast sensitivity measured with operant techniques. *Vision Res.*, **21,** 1253–66.

2 Sensory processing in human amblyopia: snakes and ladders

Robert F. Hess

INTRODUCTION

At the most general level we all know what amblyopia means; reduced and, to a greater extent, irretrievable visual capacity due to developmental causes. At another level, the most detailed, none of us knows what amblyopia is. Amblyopes are the first to admit that although their vision is reduced, for they have a fellow normal eye with which to compare, it is hard to describe exactly how it is reduced. The devil is in the detail.

It would be naïve to think that there is only one visual deficit in amblyopia. Visual processing is not only parallel in nature, it also has important bottom-up and top-down aspects. The former follows from the many separate pre-striate areas devoted to analysing different visual capacities within the same region of the visual field. The latter is reflected in the anatomical connections between different cortical as well as pre-cortical areas; the feedback from higher cortical areas is no less than the feed-forward connections.

Given this complexity, where should we start in our quest to understand amblyopia? There is no simple answer to this. I am going to suggest that a suitable starting point concerns visual perception in amblyopia. In other words, what is the dominant feature of the perceptual deficit in amblyopia? In a nutshell, what is the main reason why amblyopes find it so difficult to perform everyday tasks with their affected eye? Once we have identified this, let us chance our arm at what its neural basis might be. Historically, it's been like a game of snakes and ladders; climbing up the apparently solid ladders leading to a plausible explanation, only to slide down a snake when such an explanation is disproven.

FIRST LADDER

The first quantitative glimpse of the visual deficit in amblyopia came when Daniel Green and Roger Gstalder (Gstalder and Green, 1971) published the first contrast sensitivity function on an amblyope (Figure 2.1). Their results showed that amblyopes required more contrast to detect high spatial frequency targets. Their low spatial frequency sensitivity was normal.

Figure 2.1 *Comparison of contrast sensitivity for the normal (filled symbols) and fellow amblyopic (unfilled symbols) eye for a strabismic amblyope (from Gstalder and Green, 1971).*

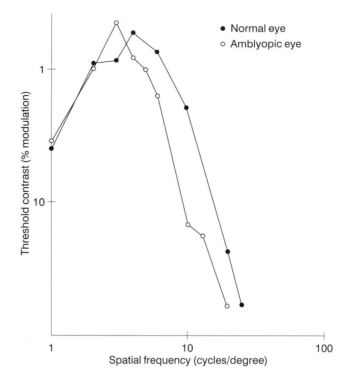

Later Hess and Howell (1977) showed that some amblyopes, in this case strabismic amblyopes, could have loss of sensitivity at low spatial frequencies as well as the high spatial frequency loss previously reported by Gstalder and Green (Figure 2.2).

At the same time, Levi and Harwerth (1977) reported similar measurements on anisometropic amblyopes. There were two puzzling things about these

Figure 2.2 *Examples of the types of contrast sensitivity losses in strabismic amblyopia. In each case, the normal (unfilled symbols) and fellow amblyopic (filled symbols) eyes are compared. In the upper frame, the ratio of sensitivity for the normal/amblyopic eye is plotted (from Hess and Howell, 1977).*

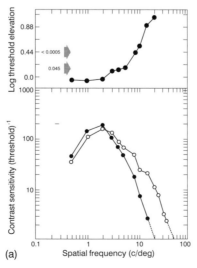

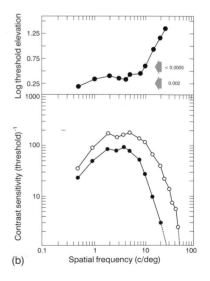

initial findings. The first was that the contrast sensitivity losses appeared to be quite mild, grating acuity being much less affected than letter acuity (Levi and Klein, 1982). This suggested that the deficit should be visually less debilitating than it appeared from the reports given by amblyopes. Secondly, strabismics and anisometropes appeared indistinguishable as seen through the contrast sensitivity viewer, yet from a clinical point of view they were seen as two quite separate entities.

FIRST SNAKE

One could be forgiven, at the time, for emphasizing the reduction in the spatial range available to the amblyopic visual system. Since optical blur results in a similar loss of acuity, it was natural to think of amblyopes as having blurred vision. The photograph that is shown in Figure 2.3a is of two prominent visual scientists who for the present will remain nameless. You can imagine that they are examining an amblyope; what we see is the view from the amblyope's perspective. This will allow me to simulate different models of the perception in amblyopia that represent different points in our evolving understanding of the condition.

In Figure 2.3b we see a simulation of what an amblyope would see if the problem were solely that of reduced acuity as quantified by the reduced spatial range covered by the contrast sensitivity measurements of the amblyopic visual system. Is amblyopia simply blurred vision? The answer is no! Amblyopes do not report that objects look more blurred when their vision is restricted to their amblyopic eyes. Jonathan Pointer and I (unpublished) verified this by asking amblyopes to make perceptual matches for edges of different sharpness shown to the normal and fellow amblyopic eyes. For example, a comparison edge of a fixed sharpness can be shown to the amblyopic eye and the amblyope can be asked to make a perceptual match with an identical edge of variable sharpness shown to the fellow normal eye. This can be repeated for comparison edges varying from very blurred to very sharp. The results for a normal subject show, unsurprisingly, that with two normal eyes, edges are matched veridically and the results fall along a 45° sloping line. In the case where one eye is optically blurred, also unsurprisingly, the more blurred one eye is the less sharp edges are perceived. Results for an anisometropic (i.e. non-strabismic) amblyope show that they also perceive sharp edges as slightly blurred by the amblyopic eye, but the magnitude of the effect is much less than one would expect from the acuity deficit. Surprisingly, results for a strabismic amblyope with a severe acuity loss show that even the sharpest edges are perceived to be sharp. This is surprising, because it does not follow from the known contrast sensitivity loss and our current understanding of how blur is signalled by the visual system. Whatever the explanation, it means that amblyopes do not have a blurred perception, and thus our understanding of amblyopia must involve more than their restricted spatial range (i.e. the acuity loss).

Figure 2.3 *(a) An original photograph of two eminent visual scientists. (b) A simulation of amblyopic perception in terms of optical blur.*

AMBLYOPIC PERCEPTION?

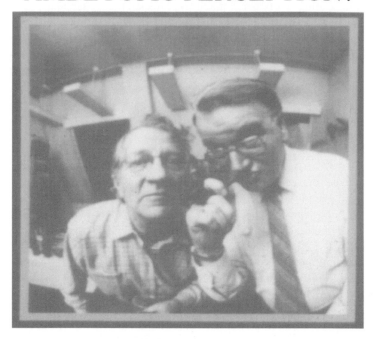

IS IT BLURRED?

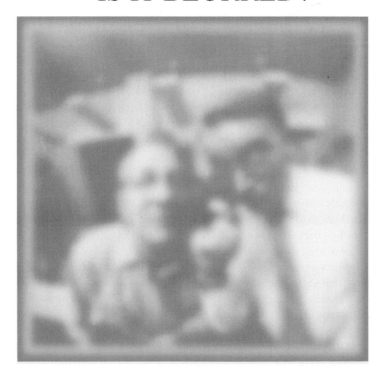

ANOTHER SNAKE

Contrast sensitivity measurements on amblyopes indicate that not only is the spatial range restricted, but also more contrast is required to detect objects which fall within the amblyope's passband. We have also seen that for some amblyopes this contrast sensitivity deficit extends to all spatial frequencies (i.e. very low spatial frequencies). Could it be that the contrast sensitivity deficit is key to amblyopia? In other words, do amblyopes perceive everyday objects at a much reduced contrast, as simulated in Figure 2.4?

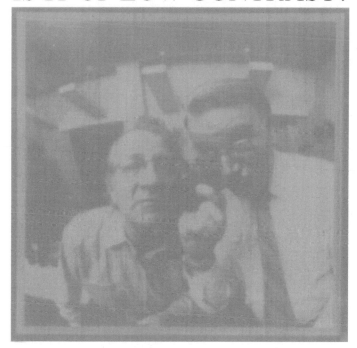

IS IT OF LOW CONTRAST?

Figure 2.4 *A simulation of amblyopic perception in terms of reduced contrast.*

One way of testing this is to ask amblyopes to match the contrast of the same object seen by each eye. Arthur Bradley and I (Hess and Bradley, 1980) asked amblyopes to match a fixed contrast stimulus presented to the amblyopic eye with a variable contrast stimulus seen by the normal eye. The stimulus was a spatial sine-wave grating of a particular spatial frequency. This can be done for a range of fixed contrasts extending from threshold to 100 per cent. Results for two amblyopes, a strabismic and a non-strabismic, are seen in Figure 2.5.

Here, we are plotting the fixed comparison contrast seen by the amblyopic eye against the variable matching contrast seen by the fellow normal eye. For a normal observer, all the results would fit along the 45° diagonal because the

Figure 2.5 *Dichoptic contrast matching results for (a) a representative strabismic and (b) a non-strabismic, anisometropic amblyope. The unfilled symbols represent contrast thresholds, and the solid sloping line, the veridical matching results expected for a normal observer (from Hess and Bradley, 1980).*

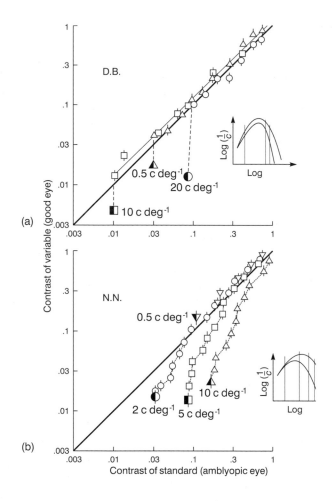

contrasts in the two eyes would be seen veridically. In the case of the strabismic (Figure 2.5a), the half-filled symbols represent the threshold points. For example, take the results for 20 c/deg; the amblyopic eye needed a contrast of 0.1 to see it, whereas the normal fellow eye required a contrast of 0.01. Thus the amblyopic eye required 10 times more contrast to detect it. However, notice that once the stimulus is just above its elevated threshold it is seen veridically, and this is maintained from threshold to 100 per cent. This suggests that although thresholds are elevated, supra-threshold contrast perception is normal. Essentially the same conclusion is arrived at for the non-strabismic amblyope, except that the process is much more gradual. Contrasts are now perceived normally not just above threshold but a fair way above threshold. Under normal viewing conditions everyday images are of quite high contrast (i.e. above 30 per cent), and in this range neither type of amblyope, on the basis of these matching results, would be expected to perceive contrast differently with their amblyopic eye. Contrast is not the main problem.

A LADDER AT LAST

Amblyopes are quick to tell you just that – namely that the perception through their amblyopic eye is neither blurred nor of less contrast. Although they can tell you what their perception isn't, they find it hard to describe exactly what it is. Using simple geometric patterns can greatly facilitate this (Hess *et al.*, 1978). Amblyopes, especially strabismic amblyopes, report severe spatial distortions for such patterns when viewing with their amblyopic eye. An example is shown in Figure 2.6 for a strabismic amblyope whose contrast sensitivity (but not their letter acuity) was normal. The reported spatial distortions are seen to vary with spatial frequency. These distortions are not fixed, and these drawings are only a very approximate description of what they see. Even given that, they do suggest that the problem may have nothing to do with the associated contrast sensitivity deficit.

There have been a number of attempts to quantify these. Merton Flom, Harold Bedell and colleagues in Houston used a spatial bisection task (Bedell and Flom, 1981, 1983; Bedell *et al.*, 1985); Ruxandra Sireteanu, Maria Fronius and colleagues in Frankfurt used a shape completion task (Fronius and Sireteanu, 1989, 1992; Lagreze and Sireteanu, 1991, 1992); Denis Levi, Stan Klein and colleagues in Houston used a vernier alignment task (Levi and Klein, 1983, 1985, 1986, 1992, 1996; Levi *et al.*, 1987, 1994). Ian Holliday and I (Hess and Holliday, 1992) used an alignment task for elements that were not only spatial frequency narrowband but also well separated in space (stimuli illustrated in Figure 2.7 in three scaled sets; small, medium and large).

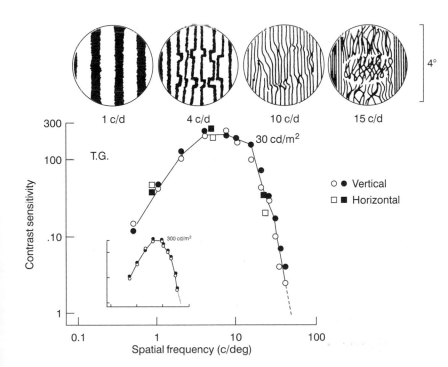

Figure 2.6 *Upper frame: drawings made by an amblyope of how grating stimuli are perceived by the amblyopic eye. Lower frame: contrast sensitivity measurements, which are normal in this case (from Hess et al., 1978).*

Figure 2.7 *Stimuli used in the three-element spatial alignment task by Hess and Holliday (1992). Three different scaled sets are displayed, each consisting of two outer reference elements (Gabors) and a central element whose alignment is judged.*

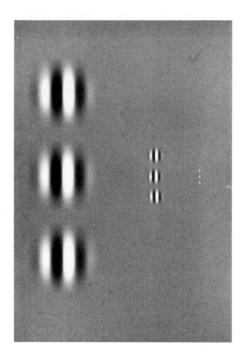

We did this for three reasons. First, we wanted a task that could not be done with single visual filters (and hence would not bear a simple relationship to the contrast sensitivity loss); second, a stimulus that would enable us to investigate how the positional deficit varied with spatial scale; and third, a stimulus that would allow us to compensate for the known contrast sensitivity loss at each of the spatial scales investigated.

We wanted to know whether the positional deficit should be best thought of in terms of fixed dimension (e.g. so many minutes of visual angle), or as a fixed proportion of the scale of the stimuli used to investigate it (which would make sense in terms of a scale space analysis). Results for a group of strabismic amblyopes are displayed in Figure 2.8.

Here, we are plotting the accuracy with which the central Gabor element (refer to Figure 2.7) can be aligned with the two fixed reference Gabors against the spatial scale of the stimuli (i.e. small, medium or large examples shown in Figure 2.7). Accuracy for the normal eye varies with the scale of the stimuli used (open symbols). The amblyopic visual system is clearly abnormal, and the extent of this abnormality does not vary with stimulus scale (results for amblyopic and normal fellow eyes are displaced parallel on these log co-ordinates). Our question is answered; the positional abnormality is scale-invariant – that is, it cannot be thought of in terms of a fixed spatial dimension for any individual amblyope (see also Demanins and Hess, 1996). The neural representation of space is equally disrupted at all scales. What this means is that the simulation shown in Figure 2.9a, where we have randomized the pixels over a fixed spatial range, is not a good model of the positional

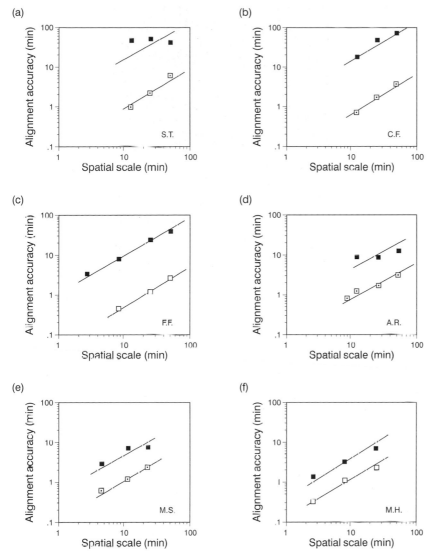

Figure 2.8 *Alignment accuracy in minutes of arc is plotted against spatial scale (see Figure 2.7) in minutes of arc for the normal (unfilled symbols) and fellow amblyopic eyes (filled symbols) of six strabismic amblyopes. The positional loss is large and scale invariant (from Hess and Holliday, 1992).*

disruption, as this affects only information at the finest scale. A better simulation is seen in Figure 2.9b, where the disruption is a constant fraction of each scale represented in the photograph; now coarse as well as fine scales are affected to the same degree.

Is this positional abnormality related to the previously described contrast sensitivity loss? In the above experiment, we ensured that the stimuli to be positioned were visible to the amblyopic eye. This was achieved by displaying the stimuli at equal multiples above threshold for the normal and amblyopic eye. Thus we have already factored out the contrast sensitivity loss. However, it still could be that both the contrast sensitivity loss and the positional loss

Figure 2.9 *(a) A simulation of positional uncertainty in terms of a pixel disarray. (b) A simulation of positional uncertainty in terms of a disarray that is proportional to spatial scale.*

DISTORTED LIKE THIS?

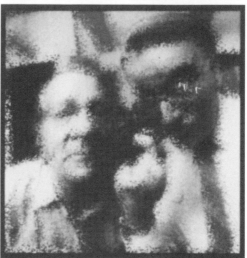

(a)

DISTORTED LIKE THIS?

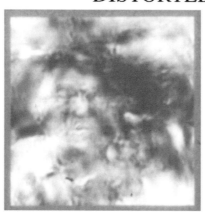 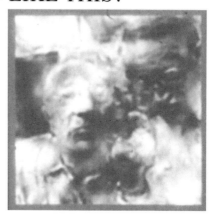

(b)

have a common cause. Figure 2.10 shows a scatter plot of the relationship between the positional and contrast sensitivity losses for a group of strabismic (open symbols) and non-strabismic, anisometropic amblyopes (filled symbols). In non-strabismic, anisometropic amblyopia there is no real evidence for a positional loss at all once the contrast sensitivity problem has been accounted for (the dashed line indicates a ratio of unity, i.e. no loss). Vernier acuity measurements which probably involve very different mechanisms also support this conclusion by exhibiting a strong correlation with grating acuity (Levi and Klein, 1985). Strabismics do exhibit significant positional losses, but these are uncorrelated with their contrast sensitivity loss. We must conclude that they represent independent deficits.

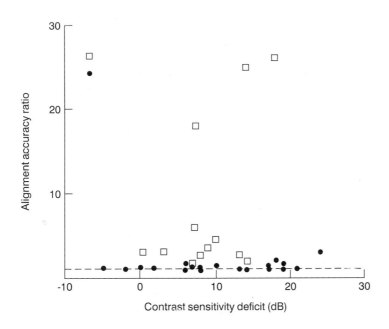

Figure 2.10 *Relationship between the deficits for positional uncertainty and contrast sensitivity in strabismic (unfilled symbols) and anisometropic (i.e. non-strabismic) amblyopes (filled symbols). The dashed line represents a ratio of unity (i.e. no deficit) (from Hess and Holliday, 1992).*

THE NATURE OF THE POSITIONAL DEFICIT

In principle, this positional deficit could be due to one of a number of causes. The most obvious ones are:

1. An under-representation of visual space by cortical cells
2. Anomalous interactions between cells that encode spatial relationships
3. A disordered or inaccurate representation of space by a normal complement of cells.

Let's look at each of these in turn.

If the problem is simply that the amblyopic cortex has fewer cells tilling the visual field, there is a straightforward prediction that there should be a correlated loss in contrast discrimination (Hess and Field, 1994). Take the example of a visual system with only one cell. Because its output is one-dimensional (i.e. univariant), it cannot know whether it was stimulated by a low contrast aligned (with respect to its peak sensitivity) target, or a high contrast misaligned target (illustrated in Figure 2.11).

Now let's consider a visual system comprising two closely spaced cells, as depicted in Figure 2.12a (top frame). The code for contrast would involve adding the outputs of these two cells. The code for position would involve subtracting the outputs. For such a simple system, the response surface can be computed in terms of iso-contrast and iso-position lines; the spacing between these contours relate to the system's accuracy for contrast and position (Figure 2.12a, bottom frame).

Figure 2.11 *An illustration of the covariation of positional and contrast errors in a univariant visual detector (from Hess and Field, 1994).*

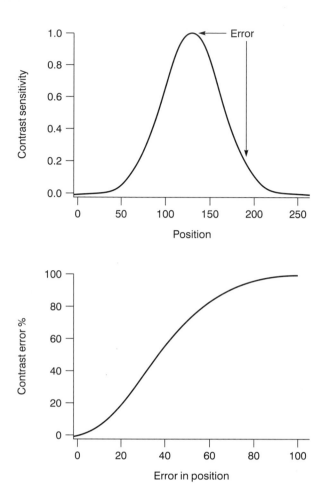

Now imagine that these detectors are more widely separated, as illustrated in Figure 2.12b (top frame). This will result in the contours for contrast and position being more closely packed, which reflects the consequent loss in accuracy for position and contrast (Figure 2.12b, bottom frame).

For a visual system with N cells, an N-dimensional space needs to be considered; however, the conclusion is the same – loss of accuracy for contrast and position when detectors are more widely spaced due to less cells. Assuming that there are not separate pathways for the encoding of contrast and for position, or that any common detectors are not extremely narrowband (Levi and Klein, 1996), then this argument holds. David Field and I (Hess and Field, 1994) used a 2×2 AFC task in which amblyopes had first to judge whether the middle element of a three-element alignment stimulus (as in Figure 2.13a) was aligned with respect to the two outer reference elements, and secondly whether it was of higher or lower contrast compared with the outer reference elements. The results are shown in Figure 2.13b; there is only a very shallow relationship between the accuracy for position and contrast.

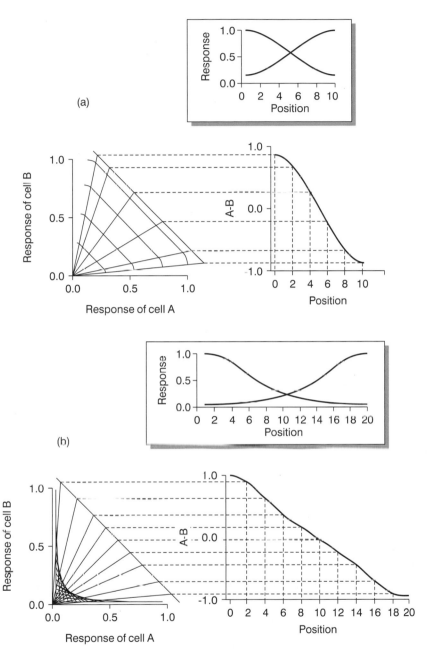

Figure 2.12 *(a) The position (dashed lines) and contrast (solid lines) response space (bottom left) for two overlapping and two closely spaced detectors for pulse-like stimuli of different contrasts and in different positions of the receptive fields. (b) The position (dashed lines) and contrast (solid lines) response space (bottom left) for two overlapping but widely spaced detectors for pulse-like stimuli of different contrasts and in different positions of the receptive fields. The sensitivity profiles are given in the upper graph, and the subtractive positional code in the lower right graph. Notice that now both the iso-position (dashed lines) and iso-contrast lines (solid lines) are closer together compared with the closely spaced detectors of (a) (from Hess and Field, 1994).*

There have been other approaches to this same issue (Hess and Anderson, 1993; Demanins *et al.*, 1999) with the same conclusion. On the other hand, Dennis Levi and collaborators (Levi and Klein, 1986; Levi *et al.*, 1987, 1994; Sharma *et al.*, 1999) have argued that under-sampling plays a major role in the amblyopic deficit, although I don't think the evidence has been overwhelming.

Figure 2.13 *(a) Stimulus for measuring thresholds for position and contrast. In a three-element alignment task, subjects are asked to decide on the position and contrast of the middle element relative to the outer two reference elements. (b) Relationship between thresholds for positional and contrast accuracy measured simultaneously in a 2 x 2 AFC paradigm in a group of strabismic amblyopes.*

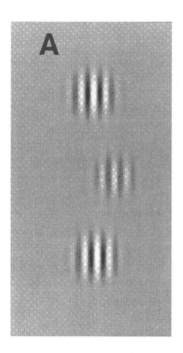

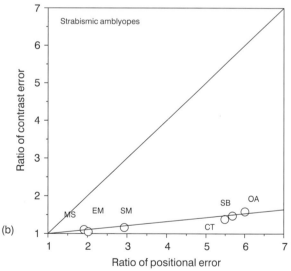

(b)

Another possibility is that the spatial distortions reported by amblyopes and their subsequently measured positional uncertainty may be due to anomalous interactions between a normal complement of cells in an otherwise normal topographical arrangement (Polat *et al.*, 1997). This is difficult to assess, simply because it is likely that what appears to be anomalous lateral interactions could equally well be due to a purely positional disruption. In other words, the cortical topography could be disrupted, but the interactions

A

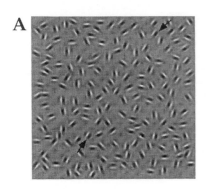

B

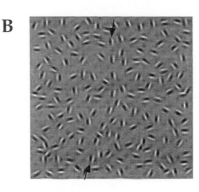

C

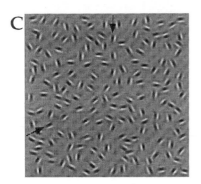

D

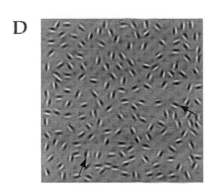

Figure 2.14 *Examples of contours of different curvature constructed from co-oriented and co-aligned Gabor elements embedded in a field of similar elements but of random position and orientation.*

between adjacent cells may be entirely normal. Let me give you a specific example. One task that has been shown to rely on lateral interactions is the contour integration paradigm (Field *et al.*, 1993). Subjects are required to detect contours composed of oriented Gabors embedded in a field of identical elements but of random orientation. Some examples of contours of different curvature are shown in Figure 2.14.

This task has been shown to depend conjointly on element position and local orientation (for a review, see Hess and Field, 1999). Amblyopes, especially strabismics, exhibit anomalous contour integration on this task even when the individual elements are well above their elevated contrast thresholds (Hess *et al.*, 1997). These results are shown in Figure 2.15, where percentage correct contour detection is plotted against contour curvature for the normal (open symbols) and fellow amblyopic eyes (filled symbols) for a group of strabismic amblyopes.

By adding orientational noise to the elements comprising the contour, it is possible to assess whether this deficit in performance is due to anomalous interactions between local orientation detectors. Figure 2.16 shows that performance for the normal and amblyopic eyes cannot be brought together by interfering with the local orientational information, and the explanation for the deficient contour integration must lie elsewhere.

Figure 2.15 *Results for contour detection in a group of strabismic amblyopes. Percent correct contour detection is plotted against the contour curvature for the normal (unfilled symbols) and fellow amblyopic eye (filled symbols) (from Hess et al., 1997).*

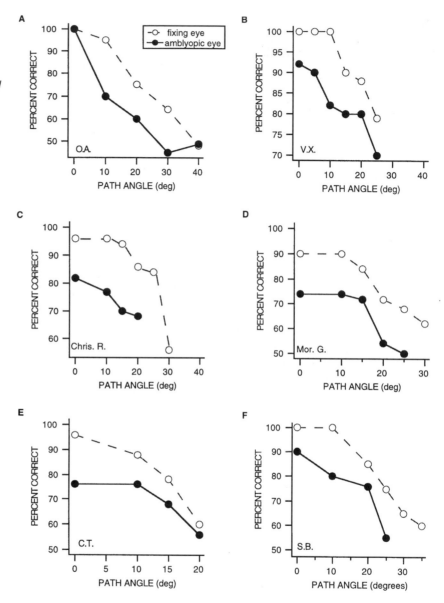

One possibility is that the deficient positional coding, which has been discussed above, could underlie the reduced performance on this task. Figure 2.17 shows that if positional noise is added to the elements of the contour then normal and amblyopic performance can be equated, suggesting a role for the positional deficit in explaining the reduced performance of amblyopes on this task.

Indeed, when the magnitude of the positional deficit is measured for each amblyope (see Hess *et al.*, 1997 for specific details) and the stimuli

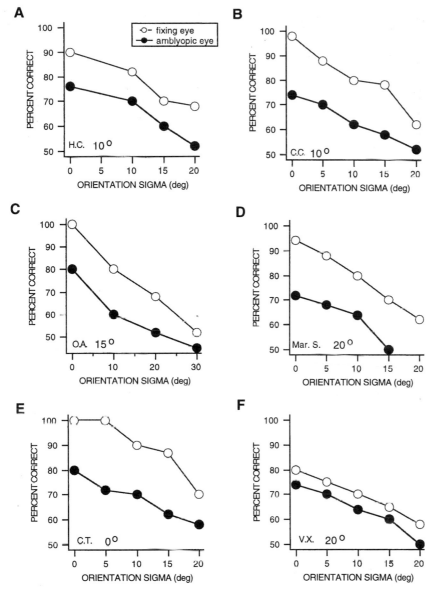

Figure 2.16 *The effect of orientational noise on contour detection for the normal (unfilled symbols) and fellow amblyopic eye (filled symbols) for contours of varying curvature (from Hess et al., 1997).*

positionally perturbed to this extent, the normal and amblyopic performance are approximately equal (see Figure 2.18).

This suggests that the reason why amblyopes exhibit anomalous contour integration is because their positional coding is disrupted, and not because of anomalous lateral interactions between orientational detectors. If there are anomalous lateral interactions in amblyopia, they must not be a general phenomenon and may be limited to positional encoding. We are left with a chicken and egg problem; does positional uncertainty result in what looks like

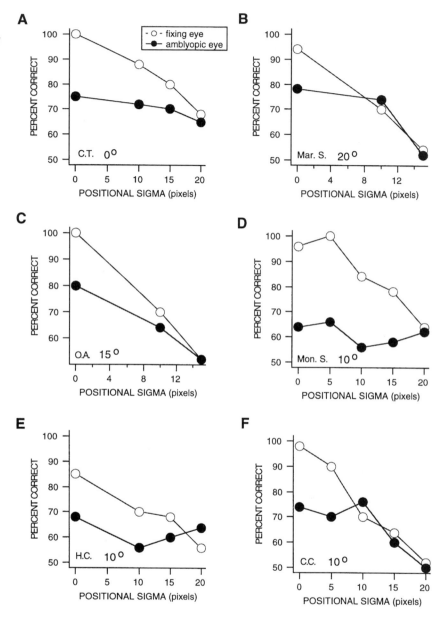

Figure 2.17 *The effect of positional noise on contour detection for the normal (unfilled symbols) and fellow amblyopic eye (filled symbols) for contours of varying curvature (from Hess et al., 1997).*

anomalous lateral interactions, or do anomalous lateral interactions result in positional uncertainty?

A POSSIBLE SNAKE

The major problem in amblyopia is positional uncertainty, yet we know so little about how we encode position – at least for well-separated elements

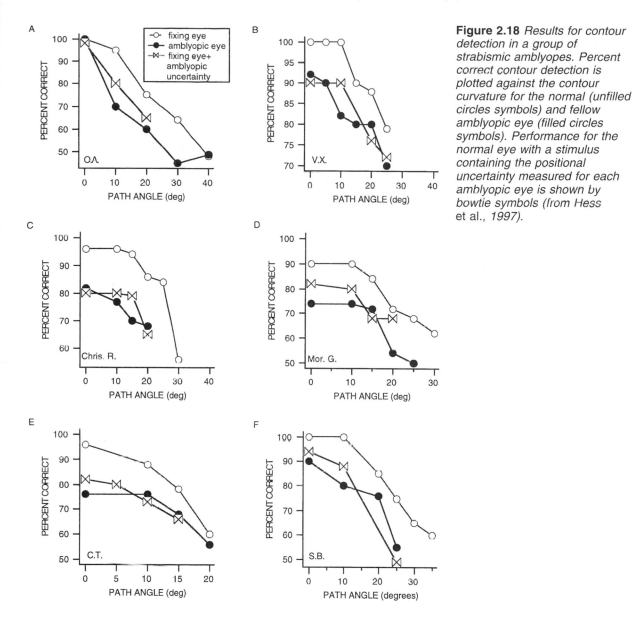

Figure 2.18 *Results for contour detection in a group of strabismic amblyopes. Percent correct contour detection is plotted against the contour curvature for the normal (unfilled circles symbols) and fellow amblyopic eye (filled circles symbols). Performance for the normal eye with a stimulus containing the positional uncertainty measured for each amblyopic eye is shown by bowtie symbols (from Hess et al., 1997).*

where local luminance, local contrast and local orientation can provide powerful but indirect clues to position. Is positional accuracy a reflection of 'bottom-up' or 'top-down' processing? It has always been assumed that it represents a bottom-up process, but there is no hard evidence to support this assertion. If it depends on top-down influences, then the deficit in amblyopia may implicate the extensive feedback pathways from extra-striate to striate cortex, rather than the traditional feed-forward ones.

AT LEAST TWO TYPES OF AMBLYOPIA

We generally talk about amblyopia as a single entity, but there is now ample evidence to suggest that strabismic and non-strabismic forms may be different. I have already mentioned three important differences; blur perception, contrast perception and positional accuracy. In each of these, there are quantitative differences between strabismic and non-strabismic amblyopes. Let me now add a further, and I believe important, difference that involves how the contrast threshold loss is distributed across the visual field. In Figure 2.19, results are displayed for a single representative strabismic and non-strabismic amblyope (from the results of Hess *et al.*, 1980).

In Figure 2.20, results are given for a population of strabismic and non-strabismic amblyopes (Hess and Pointer, 1985). In Figure 2.19, we are comparing the contrast sensitivity deficit by plotting the ratio of sensitivity (termed 'threshold elevation') as a function of spatial frequency. This is done for two different targets; a purely central one and a purely peripheral one. In the case of the strabismic, there is a sizeable contrast sensitivity deficit for the central target that increases with spatial frequency. Notice that this deficit all

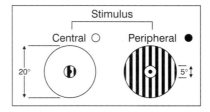

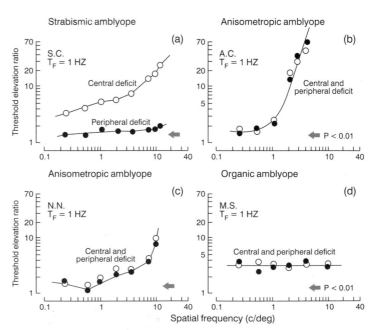

Figure 2.19 *Comparison of the contrast sensitivity deficit for a purely foveal and a purely peripheral stimulus (top frame) for a representative strabismic and anisometropic (i.e. non-strabismic) amblyope (from Hess et al., 1980).*

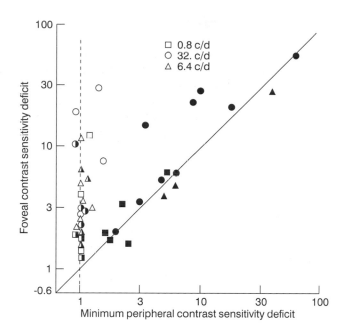

Figure 2.20 *Relationship between the foveal and peripheral deficits for contrast sensitivity in a group of purely strabismic (unfilled symbols), purely anisometropic (filled symbols), and mixed strabismic/anisometropic (half-filled symbols) amblyopes (from Hess and Pointer, 1985).*

but disappears when the peripheral target is used (ratios now hover just above unity). The contrast sensitivity deficit is mainly centrally located in the visual field. Compare this with the situation for the non-strabismic anisometrope. Here the contrast sensitivity deficit, which is even more severe than for the strabismic, is uninfluenced by whether we use a central or peripheral stimulus, suggesting that the underlying deficit is rather evenly distributed across the visual field. For a population of amblyopes (Figure 2.20) we now have two different predictions; either the deficit is evenly distributed across the visual field (the solid sloping line in Figure 2.20), or it just involves the fovea (the vertical, dashed line in Figure 2.20). The filled symbols refer to the non-strabismic anisometropes, the open symbols to the strabismics, and the half-filled symbols to the strabismic anisometropes. The foveal deficit is plotted against the minimum peripheral deficit. The minimum peripheral deficit is used because there are sizeable asymmetries seen in the region loss in strabismic amblyopia (Hess and Pointer, 1985). The results divide along the lines of whether a strabismus is present or not; in the former case the deficit is mainly foveal, whereas in the latter case it is more evenly distributed across the visual field. With all these differences between strabismic and non-strabismic amblyopia, it is hard to accept that amblyopia is a single entity; surely there must be at least two?

A SNAKE: ANIMAL MODELS

Animal models of human amblyopia have told us very little about the possible neural basis of the above deficits. What they have told us is limited to the contrast sensitivity deficit, which does not lie at the heart of the amblyopes perceptual disability. In general, the animal models have come to two main conclusions: there is no difference between strabismic and non-strabismic anisometropic amblyopia, and the sole deficit in amblyopia is contrast sensitivity (see Kiorpes and McKee, 1999). Both of these conclusions are at odds with the bulk of the psychophysics of human amblyopia as outlined in this chapter. Either the way amblyopia is produced in these models is inappropriate, or the tools that are used to assess vision are less than ideal. I favour the latter explanation; measures of positional accuracy that rely on vernier-like tasks are open to the criticism that local luminance/contrast /orientation is used *indirectly* to code position (Carney and Klein, 1999). In such a case it would be expected that contrast sensitivity would set the limit to performance (accuracy strongly depends on contrast), as it is another reflection of the same sensitivity. In the positional measures described above using well-separated Gabors, contrast sensitivity cannot account for the reduced positional performance of strabismic amblyopes (accuracy only weakly depends on contrast). Those involved in animal models have to come to grips with this finding. Recent reports (Gingras *et al.*, 1999) in strabismic cats suggest that, using an identical task with well-separated Gabors, there are profound positional uncertainty deficits that completely overshadow the previously described acuity and contrast sensitivity losses. One of the fundamental criticisms of the animal modelling approach is that once the problem goes beyond anomalies to individual cells, the techniques are not well established to assess it. Positional uncertainty *per se* is one such case. There are no current models of how we encode position within a neuronal population, and no current techniques to assess a possible deficit in an animal made artificially amblyopic. Until we advance beyond this current limit, animal models may have little to say about the main deficit in amblyopia.

A POSSIBLE LADDER

The positional deficit in amblyopia has exclusively been considered in terms of a low-level sensory deficit. The problem has always been how position is encoded in the outputs of cortical cells early in the pathway. No cells have been found in the striate cortex whose output encodes position *per se*. It is possible that the positional framework is provided by a top-down attentional mechanism. Support for this comes from some current experiments that Steven Dakin, Gareth Barnes, Serge Dumoulin and I are doing, which show that our capacity for extracting positional information is very limited; we are accurate at telling the relative position of one element, but very poor at telling the relative position of two elements. It is as if we have only two position tags, one for a test object and another for a reference. During saccadic eye movements our space perception is disrupted (Ross *et al.*, 1997), and this could be due to a transient disruption to such a higher-level attentional mechanism, whose normal job is to provide the framework for spatial position. The most likely location for this processing, based on what we presently know, is the prefrontal cortex. The 'what' and 'where' pathways (Ungerleider and Mishkin, 1982) are kept separate up to this point (Logothetis, 1998). There is evidence that in the prefrontal cortex, cells show both spatial and object tuning (Rao *et al.*, 1997). If the top-down, attentional model that I have advanced is correct, the positional deficit may well lie even at this late stage in the pathway.

ACKNOWLEDGEMENTS

I gratefully acknowledge the contribution made by all my colleagues, not just those named in this review, and for the support of the Medical Research Council of Canada.

REFERENCES

Bedell, H. D. and Flom, M. C. (1981). Monocular spatial distortion in strabismic amblyopia. *Inv. Ophthalmol. Vis. Sci.*, **20**, 263–8.

Bedell, H. E. and Flom, M. C. (1983). Normal and abnormal space perception. *Am. J. Optom. Physiol. Optics*, **60**, 426–35.

Bedell, H. E., Flom, M. C. and Barbeito, R. (1985). Spatial aberrations and acuity in strabismus and amblyopia. *Inv. Ophthalmol. Vis. Sci.*, **26**, 909–16.

Carney, T. and Klein, S. A. (1999). Optimum spatial localization is limited by contrast sensitivity. *Vision Res.*, **39**, 503–11.

Demanins, R. and Hess, R. F. (1996). Positional loss in strabismic amblyopia – interrelationship of alignment threshold, bias, spatial scale and eccentricity. *Vision Res.*, **36**, 2771–94.

Demanins, R., Wang, Y.-Z. and Hess, R. F. (1999). The neural deficit in strabismic amblyopia: sampling considerations. *Vision Res.*, **39**, 3575–85.

Field, D. J., Hayes, A. and Hess, R. F. (1993). Contour integration by the human visual system: evidence for a local 'association field'. *Vision Res.*, **33**, 173–93.

Fronius, M. and Sireteanu, R. (1989). Monocular geometry is selectively distorted in the central visual field of strabismic amblyopes. *Inv. Ophthalmol. Vis. Sci.*, **30**, 2034–44.

Fronius, M. and Sireteanu, R. (1992). Localization disorders in squint amblyopia: horizontal line bisection and relative vertical localization. *Klin. Monats. Augenheilk.*, **201**, 22–9.

Gingras, G., Mitchell, D. E. and Hess, R. F. (1999). The spatial localization deficit in visually deprived kittens. *Inv. Ophthalmol. Vis. Sci.*, **40**, S54.

Polat, U., Sagi, D. and Norcia, A. M. (1997). Abnormal long-range spatial interactions in amblyopia. *Vision Res.*, **37**, 737–44.

Gstalder, R. J. and Green, D. G. (1971). Laser interferometric acuity in amblyopia. *J. Ped. Ophthalmol.*, **8**, 251–6.

Hess, R. F. and Anderson, S. J. (1993). Motion sensitivity and spatial undersampling in amblyopia. *Vision Res.*, **33**, 881–96.

Hess, R. F. and Bradley, A. (1980). Contrast coding in amblyopia is only minimally impaired above threshold. *Nature (Lond.)*, **287**, 463–4.

Hess, R. F. and Field, D. J. (1994). Is the spatial deficit in strabismic amblyopia due to loss of cells or an uncalibrated disarray of cells? *Vision Res.*, **34**, 3397–406.

Hess, R. F. and Field, D. J. (1999). Contour integration: new insights. *Trends Cognitive Sci.*, **3**, 480–86.

Hess, R. F. and Holliday, I. E. (1992). The spatial localization deficit in amblyopia. *Vision Res.*, **32**, 1319–39.

Hess, R. F. and Howell, E. R. (1977). The threshold contrast sensitivity function in strabismic amblyopia: evidence for a two type classification. *Vision Res.*, **17**, 1049–55.

Hess, R. F. and Pointer, J. S. (1985). Differences in the neural basis of human amblyopias: the distribution of the anomaly across the visual field. *Vision Res.*, **25**, 1577–94.

Hess, R. F., Campbell, F. W. and Greenhalgh, T. (1978). On the nature of the neural abnormality in human amblyopia; neural aberrations and neural sensitivity loss. *Pflugers Archiv – Eur. J. Physiol.*, **377**, 201–7.

Hess, R. F., Campbell, F. W. and Zimmern, R. (1980). Differences in the neural basis of human amblyopias: effect of mean luminance. *Vision Res.*, **20**, 295–305.

Hess, R. F., McIllhagga, W. and Field, D. J. (1997). Contour integration in strabismic amblyopia: the sufficiency of an explanation based on positional uncertainty. *Vision Res.*, **37**, 3145–61.

Kiorpes, L. and McKee, S. P. (1999). Neural mechanisms underlying amblyopia. *Curr. Opin. Neurobiol.*, **9**, 480–86.

Lagreze, W. D. and Sireteanu, R. (1991). Two-dimensional spatial distortions in human strabismic amblyopia. *Vision Res.*, **31**, 1271–88.

Lagreze, W. D. and Sireteanu, R. (1992). Errors of monocular localization in strabismic amblyopia. Two-dimensional distortion. *Klin. Monats. Augenheilk.*, **201**, 92–6.

Levi, M. and Harwerth, R. S. (1977). Spatio-temporal interactions in anisometropic and strabismic amblyopia. *Inv. Ophthalmol. Vis. Sci.*, **16**, 90–95.

Levi, D. M. and Klein, S. (1982). Hyperacuity and amblyopia. *Nature (Lond.)*, **298**, 268–70.

Levi, D. M. and Klein, S. A. (1983). Spatial localization in normal and amblyopic vision. *Vision Res.*, **23**, 1005–17.

Levi, D. M. and Klein, S. A. (1985). Vernier acuity, crowding and amblyopia. *Vision Res.*, **25**, 979–91.

Levi, D. M. and Klein, S. A. (1986). Sampling in spatial vision. *Nature*, **320**, 360–62.

Levi, D. M. and Klein, S. A. (1992). The role of local contrast in the visual deficits of humans with naturally occurring amblyopia. *Neurosci. Lett.*, **136**, 63–6.

Levi, D. M. and Klein, S. A. (1996). Limitations on position coding imposed by undersampling and univariance. *Vision Res.*, **36**, 2111–20.

Levi, D. M., Klein, S. A. and Yap, Y. L. (1987). Positional uncertainty in peripheral and amblyopic vision. *Vision Res.*, **27**, 581–97.

Levi, D. M., Klein, S. A. and Wang, H. (1994). Amblyopic and peripheral vernier acuity: a test-pedestal approach. *Vision Res.*, **34**, 3265–92.

Logothetis, N. (1998). Object vision and visual awareness. *Curr. Opin. Neurobiol.*, **8**, 536–44.

Rao, S. C., Rainer, G. and Miller, E. K. (1997). Integration of what and where in the primate prefrontal cortex. *Science*, **276**, 821–4.

Ross, J., Morrone, M. and Burr, D. C. (1997). Compression of visual space before saccades. *Nature (Lond.)*, **384**, 598–601.

Sharma, V., Levi, D. M. and Coletta, N. J. (1999). Sparse sampling of gratings in the visual cortex of strabismic amblyopes. *Vision Res.*, **39**, 3526–36.

Ungerleider, L. G. and Mishkin, M. (1982). Two cortical visual systems. In: *Analysis of Visual Behavour* (D. J. Ingle, ed.), pp. 549–86. MIT Press.

3 Functional neuroimaging in amblyopia

Stephen J. Anderson

INTRODUCTION

Historically there have been two main approaches to understanding cortical function in amblyopia: single cell studies on animals, and behavioural studies on animals and humans. Given that the sensory brain is organized into functionally discrete areas, a measure of cortical function that falls somewhere between these two approaches should be useful – in other words, a technique that provides a measure of neural activity from groups of cells with similar functional properties. Today, there are various techniques for investigating human brain function that purport to do just that. They include positron emission tomography (PET), functional magnetic resonance imaging (fMRI) and magneto-encephalography (MEG).

Ideally, one would like to see good general agreement between the animal research and the functional imaging work on humans. Sometimes this is the case. For example, the functional analysis of area MT in monkeys (Zeki, 1974; Van Essen et al., 1981) is similar to that of the homologous area V5 in humans (Zeki et al., 1991; Tootel et al., 1995; Anderson et al., 1996). However, research on amblyopia has proved to be more troublesome. Not only is there discord between the animal and human work, there is also no agreement between the various neuroimaging studies. Single cell studies on amblyopic animals have shown repeatedly that the primary visual cortex (area V1) is dysfunctional (e.g. Crewther and Crewther, 1990; Kiorpes et al., 1998; for reviews see Blakemore, 1990; Movshon and Kiorpes, 1990). However, recent PET studies on human amblyopes suggested that V1 function may be normal (Imamura et al., 1997), though earlier PET studies suggested it was abnormal (Demer et al., 1988). There is also no agreement between the fMRI studies on humans, again some suggesting V1 is normal (Sireteanu et al., 1998) and others suggesting it is abnormal (Barnes et al., 1999, 2001). My own MEG studies on strabismic adults provide evidence that V1 is dysfunctional (Anderson and Holliday, 1998; Anderson et al., 1999).

In this chapter I hope to provide a coherent explanation for these disparate results, and in so doing determine whether or not area V1 is the earliest site of dysfunction within the amblyopic visual system of humans. My conclusions are based largely on the results obtained using MEG. Before detailing this work, I include here a brief review of the major operational principles of PET, fMRI and MEG. This is done in order to demonstrate some of the more significant advantages and disadvantages of each technique, and to help explain under what circumstances they may yield different results in the assessment of amblyopia. Unless otherwise indicated, the results reported in this chapter refer to strabismic amblyopia.

REVIEW OF NEUROIMAGING TECHNIQUES

The modern era of medical imaging began in the early 1970s with the development of X-ray computed tomography (CT scans). This technique takes advantage of the fact that the amount of X-ray energy absorbed by a tissue is dependent on its density. However, the creation of a brain image using X-rays requires an enormous amount of data and sophisticated algorithms to organize it as a coherent picture. What was novel about CT scans was the use of computers to process the data and create brain images in three dimensions. This remains a valued clinical tool, but provides only structural information. PET, fMRI and MEG all provide functional information, and their basic operational principles are described below. For more general information about these techniques, the reader is referred to Aine (1995), Orrison *et al.* (1995), Toga and Mazziotta (1996) and Logothetis *et al.* (2001).

Positron emission tomography

PET requires an intravenous injection of a short-lived radioactively labelled substance, usually water for the study of tissue blood flow. The radioisotopes accumulate in the brain and emit positrons as they decay. Each positron rapidly loses energy and within a short distance ($< 5\,\text{mm}$) annihilates with an electron in the brain tissue. The burst of energy that results forms 'back-to-back' gamma rays, i.e. two gamma rays travelling along a straight line in opposite directions from the point of annihilation. These escape the body and are detected almost simultaneously by sensors on opposite sides of the patient's head. Near-simultaneous detection of gamma rays by a pair of sensors is signalled by a coincidence unit built into the circuitry of a PET scanner. The location of each ray is recorded and used to define a line of response through the brain along which the annihilation took place (Figure 3.1). Using standard reconstruction algorithms, lines of response from many different angles are counted and combined to create an image of the blood flow in the brain. To the extent that each positron emission and associated annihilation event are spatially coincident, this blood flow image reflects the spatial distribution of the radioisotopes that have been injected.

Two PET images are measured, one during a 'control' state and one during a 'task' state. The resulting images are subtracted to identify where there is extra blood flow during the task state. The major assumption is that changes in cerebral blood flow necessitated by the task reflect changes in neural activity. The disadvantages of PET include the following:

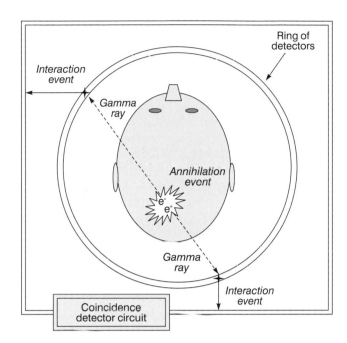

Figure 3.1 *Back-to-back gamma rays are produced when a positron (e⁺) annihilates with an electron (e⁻) in the brain tissue. The gamma rays interact with detector units in a PET scanner, allowing the exact location of each ray to be recorded. Near-simultaneous interactions are signalled using a coincidence circuit, which requires that two gamma rays be detected on opposite sides of the head within a short time interval. See text for further explanation.*

1. It is an invasive procedure in that it requires an injection of a radioisotope
2. The half-life of the radioisotope is necessarily brief, preventing a full parametric investigation of the cortical area
3. There are strict limitations on the repeated use of subjects
4. It has poor temporal resolution
5. Because of the enormous variation in human brain anatomy, its already poor spatial resolution is often made worse by the need to pool data from several subjects to enhance the signal-to-noise ratio
6. It relies on the experimental strategy of 'paired image subtraction', and therefore any conclusions drawn are dependent on the control state used
7. It assumes there is a close relationship between local neuronal activity and local blood flow.

While the latter may be true (Hartshorne, 1995), it should be kept in mind that many cells in the brain have roles other than neuronal activity – such as glial cells, which provide structural and metabolic support for the nervous system. At present there is no information on glial contributions to the PET (or fMRI) haemodynamic response.

Functional magnetic resonance imaging

MRI gives a detailed picture of the structure of the brain. This technique relies on the fact that the nuclei of atoms behave like small bar magnets. For imaging purposes, the proton nucleus of the hydrogen atom (^{1}H) is of prime importance because of its strong signal and natural abundance in brain tissue. In a normal environment the magnetic orientations of nuclei are random, and as such the brain is unmagnetized. However, when a patient's head is placed in a static magnetic field the nuclei tend to orientate either with the applied field (low energy state) or against it (high energy state). Slightly more nuclei tend to align with the field, rendering the brain weakly magnetized in this direction. Application of a radio-frequency (RF) pulse increases the proportion of nuclei aligned against the direction of the main field. When the pulse is switched off, the nuclei return to their original state and in so doing emit detectable RF signals themselves. To create an image of the brain it is necessary that the returning signals from different locations be distinguished. This can be accomplished by adding a magnetic field gradient to the main field, which has the effect of varying the frequency of the returning signals along the direction of the gradient. This procedure is called frequency encoding, and forms the basis of MRI. Of note, MRI has the advantage of being able to manipulate the contrast between different tissues by altering the RF pulses and gradients.

Importantly, the returning RF signals are affected by the chemical environment of the atoms, and it is this feature of the MRI signal that is especially important for *functional* imaging (fMRI). In brief, the amount of oxygen delivered to an active neural area exceeds that required for neural activity, resulting in a net increase in intravascular oxyhaemoglobin. The amount of oxygen carried by haemoglobin affects its magnetic properties, and MRI is sensitive to these small magnetic changes (Ogawa *et al.*, 1990). The technique is termed 'blood oxygenation level dependent' (BOLD) imaging. By comparing 'control' and 'task' states, as with PET, an image of the functionally active area can be obtained. The advantages of this technique include the following:

1. It is non-invasive, having no known biological risk
2. It provides both anatomical and functional data on each subject
3. It has excellent spatial resolution (<2 mm).

The main disadvantages are:

1. It has poor temporal resolution
2. Subject-movement artefacts can degrade the image (Hajnal *et al.*, 1994)
3. Subjects with ferromagnetic surgical implants cannot have an MRI
4. As with PET, it assumes a close relationship between local blood flow and neural activity.

Magneto-encephalography

The electrical current in the brain associated with neural activity can be measured at the surface of the head with millisecond temporal resolution using scalp electrodes. This is called electroencephalography (EEG), and it has been used for several decades to investigate brain function. Both spontaneous (e.g. alpha rhythm) and event-related (e.g. visual evoked potentials) neuroelectric activity can be measured. The latter rely on signal-averaging techniques and can be used to assess the functional organization of the brain. Unfortunately, however, electrical currents are distorted by the brain tissue and skull, making it difficult to determine the site of cortical activity. Nonetheless, electrical recordings of brain activity continue to provide valuable clinical information.

Electrical current flow in individuals produces magnetic fields that can be measured outside the body using extremely sensitive devices called magnetometers. Early research concentrated on the human heart, but technological advances have enabled the much smaller magnetic fields generated by brain activity to be recorded. This is a remarkable achievement, as the strength of the magnetic field emerging from the human brain is about 10 million times smaller than that in a typical urban environment (Figure 3.2). This technique is called magneto-encephalography (MEG), which, when combined with MRI, forms a functional image of the brain. As with EEG, both spontaneous and event-related signals can be recorded. The magnetic field emerges from the head, and induces current within the wire loops of detection coils. These are coupled to Superconducting QUantum Interference Devices (SQUIDs), which operate at liquid helium temperatures and are in essence extremely sensitive current-to-voltage converters. To reduce the level of background noise, all measurements need to be completed in a magnetically shielded room. Like EEG, MEG has excellent temporal resolution. However, as magnetic fields are little distorted by brain tissue or bone, its main advantage over electrical measures is in determining the site of cortical activity. By modelling the measured field pattern, it is possible to determine the location of the active cell population to within a few millimetres (see later, 'Neural site of amblyopic MEG response').

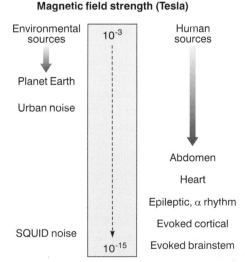

Figure 3.2 *Comparison of the strength of magnetic fields produced by human and environmental sources. (Sources: CTF MEG Systems Inc., www.ctf.com; Lewine and Orrison, 1995.)*

The advantages of MEG include the following:

1. Extracranial magnetic fields reflect neural activity (see below for details)
2. Extensive measurements can be completed on a single subject to obtain high signal-to-noise ratios, thus avoiding the need to average across subjects
3. Magnetic signals can be recorded on a time scale that is compatible with brain physiology, making it possible to resolve adjacent visual areas on the basis of their time course of activation (Aine *et al.*, 1995)
4. Unlike electrical fields, magnetic fields are not distorted by brain tissue or bone and therefore the measured magnetic fields are directly related to the primary neural sources
5. It is non-invasive.

The main disadvantage of MEG is that it does not provide any anatomical information: it is necessary to complete an MRI on each subject and co-register this data with the MEG responses.

The neurophysiological basis of MEG

As action potentials are the largest signals generated by neurons, one might suppose that they give rise to a detectable extracranial magnetic field. In fact they probably contribute little to the recorded field, principally because there is little synchronous activity across nearby axons (Lewine and Orrison, 1995). The main source of the externally recorded field is believed to be current flow associated with postsynaptic potentials (Romani *et al.*, 1982; Hämäläinen *et al.*, 1993). There are three currents to consider: current flow within the dendrite (intracellular current), which causes an outwardly directed current across the membrane (transmembrane current), which in turn produces a current around the dendrite (extracellular volume current). Of these, the transmembrane current contributes little to the external field because it is radially symmetric and the field generated by it is self-cancelling.

The dendritic field pattern of the neuron is critical in determining whether or not it contributes to the MEG signal. Neurons with circularly symmetric fields, such as stellate cells, contribute little because the symmetrical pattern of dendritic currents leads to self-cancelling magnetic fields. On the other hand, the asymmetric dendritic field pattern of pyramidal cells yields non-cancelling fields. It is generally accepted that the recorded MEG signal mostly reflects the dendritic currents of pyramidal cells.

It is thought that at least one million synapses must be synchronously active in order for an external magnetic (or electric) signal to be detectable (Martin, 1998). Although this degree of synchronous activity is possible, the geometrical considerations described above for a single cell apply equally well to a group of cells. Thus, if the asymmetric dendritic fields of pyramidal cells were arranged in a spherically symmetric fashion, no external magnetic field would be generated because of mutual cancellation of the magnetic fields associated with individual cells. This is the arrangement encountered in many subcortical structures (Lewine and Orrison, 1995). However, the dendritic fields of pyramidal cells are oriented perpendicular to the surface of the cortex and over a given region are parallel to one another, allowing synchronous activity to be recorded.

One reported difficulty with MEG is that neurons oriented radially to the scalp, such as those lying within gyri, will not give rise to an external magnetic field (Figure 3.3). This is so because in a spherical conducting

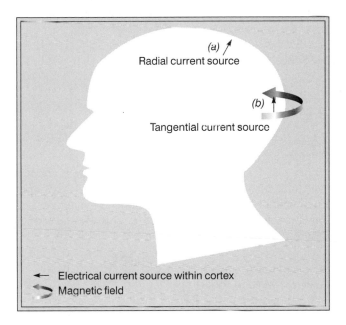

Figure 3.3 *Extracranial magnetic field generated by electrical current flow associated with neural activity.*

medium the magnetic fields generated by intra- and extracellular currents cancel each other for radially oriented cells. The standard solution to this problem is to record both MEG and EEG signals, as the latter are sensitive to radial sources. In our experience, however, we have not found 'silent sources' to be a significant problem with MEG recordings. There are at least three reasons for this:

1. The human head is not a perfectly spherical conductor
2. About 70 per cent of nerve cells lie within sulci (Van Essen and Drury, 1997; Le Goualher *et al.*, 1999), where the majority of sources have a tangential (or nearly tangential) orientation to the scalp (Hillebrand, 2000)
3. Over 50 per cent of gyral sources are non-radial by 40 degrees or more and, because of their proximity to the skull surface, are likely to produce a measurable external magnetic field (Hillebrand, 2000). This may explain why we are able to record magnetic signals from the occipital pole of amblyopes (Anderson *et al.*, 1999), where presumably many of the neurons contributing to the signal lie within the occipital gyrus.

NEUROIMAGING STUDIES ON HUMAN AMBLYOPIA

Although extensive documentation exists on the perceptual deficits in human amblyopia (see Hess *et al.*, 1990 for a review), the site and nature of the cortical deficits underlying them remain unclear. Most of our information is based on animal studies where amblyopia has been induced following either surgical or optical intervention. Even though the relationship between experimentally induced and naturally occurring amblyopia remains controversial, it is generally accepted from the animal work that the primary visual cortex is dysfunctional.

Only recently have neuroimaging tools been used to provide direct evidence of cortical dysfunction in human amblyopia. It is curious – some might say disheartening – that these studies have not yielded a coherent story.

PET

The earliest neuroimaging studies on amblyopia were completed by Demer *et al.* (1988) using PET. They examined two deprivation amblyopes, one anisometropic amblyope and one strabismic amblyope. All had a monocular acuity deficit of 6/60 or less. Their stimulus was a non-patterned stroboscopic light, flashing at a temporal frequency of 8 Hz. The level of cortical activity observed in area V1 following monocular stimulation of each subject's amblyopic eye was reduced in comparison with their normal-eye responses. However, the interocular difference in cortical activation was small, and varied between subjects. While supporting the hypothesis that area V1 is dysfunctional in amblyopia, the Demer and co-workers study has been criticized for poor statistical evaluation of the data (Imamura *et al.*, 1997) and for using inappropriate stimuli to assess cortical activity (Demer, 1993).

The PET studies of Imamura *et al.* (1997) assessed eight strabismic adults with severe amblyopia using achromatic checkerboard patterns and monocular visual stimulation. The patterns were 12.3 deg wide with a periodicity of 1.5–3.6 c/deg. Stimulation of either the normal or amblyopic eye of each subject yielded significant increases in cerebral blood flow to Brodmann's area 17 (area V1). Reduced levels of blood flow with stimulation of the amblyopic eye were only evident for extrastriate visual areas (Brodmann's areas 18 and 19). They concluded that the distorted vision of human amblyopes relates to cortical deactivation in extrastriate visual areas. Imamura and co-workers noted that their results were consistent with reports that the pattern of ocular dominance columns in human area V1 appears normal in both anisometropic (Horton and Stryker, 1993) and strabismic (Horton and Hocking, 1996) amblyopia.

fMRI

The fMRI studies of Sireteanu *et al.* (1998) also suggested that cortical activity within area V1 is normal in human amblyopia. They used sinusoidal grating stimuli of periodicity 0.5–16 c/deg and showed that, for both strabismic (four subjects) and anisometropic (five subjects) adults, monocular stimulation of the amblyopic eye always yielded reliable brain activation in area V1. They reported that the magnitude of cortical activity in areas V2, V3 and V5 was inversely correlated with the depth of amblyopia, as indicated by the psychophysically determined contrast thresholds for the detection of grating stimuli. Sireteanu and co-workers concluded that the neural deficit in human amblyopia is first apparent in area V2, becoming more pronounced at higher cortical levels.

In sharp contrast to these studies, the fMRI data of Barnes *et al.* (1999, 2001) provided evidence that cortical area V1 is affected in amblyopia. They assessed 10 strabismic adults with severe amblyopia (acuity deficit of 6/60 or less) using radial sinusoidal test patterns of 50 per cent contrast. The patterns were 5.4 degrees wide, temporally modulated at 8 Hz and viewed monocularly with central fixation. The spatial frequency of the gratings was set well below the psychophysically determined grating acuity of each subject. The site of cortical activation was similar for both normal- and amblyopic-eye viewing: activity was focused on the occipital pole near the base of the calcarine sulcus, consistent with mapping of the central visual field in area V1. In comparison with the responses driven by the normal eye, those driven by the amblyopic eye were always depressed. Barnes and co-workers concluded that area V1 is dysfunctional in human amblyopia.

Visual evoked potential

There have of course been numerous visual evoked potential (VEP) studies showing evidence of cortical dysfunction in amblyopia, several claiming that area V1 is affected (see Regan, 1989, for a review). However, as already noted, attempts to determine the site of dysfunction with electrical measures of brain activity are notoriously difficult. Moreover, much of the early VEP work was done using a small number of electrodes, making it impossible to determine with any accuracy the spatial location of cortical signals.

That said, some VEP studies have proved fruitful in understanding which cortical pathways might be affected in amblyopia. For example, Kubova *et al.* (1996) suggested that the magnocellular (M) pathway might be relatively spared in amblyopia. They used small-check patterns, stimulation being restricted to various parts of the visual field (peripheral Vs central vision, full field Vs foveal). They measured a pattern reversal VEP, where the checks were slowly counterphased at 1 Hz; and a motion onset VEP, where the checks moved rightwards at 6 deg/s. Using pattern-reversal stimulation, the amplitude of the signals from the amblyopic eye were significantly reduced under all display configurations. Moreover, the extent to which amplitude was reduced correlated well with the reduction in visual acuity (see Figure 3.4). They attributed these signals to striate activity, though no attempts were made at source localization. With motion onset there was little or no difference between the normal- and amblyopic-eye responses. They postulated that the motion-onset responses arose from an extra-striate motion area and concluded

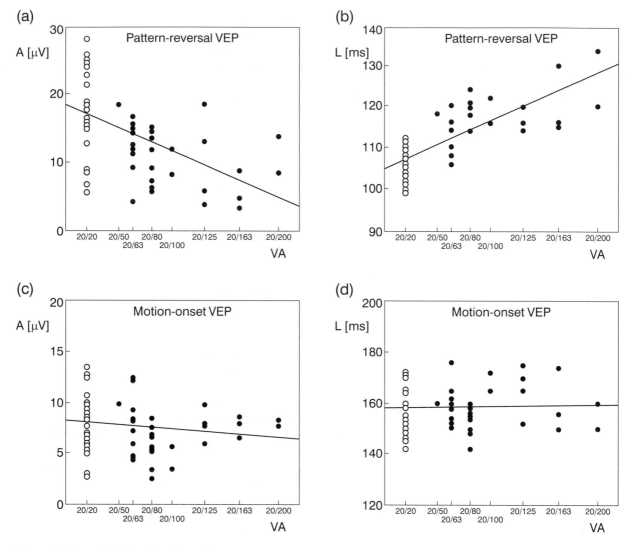

Figure 3.4 *Amplitude (a, c) and latency (b, d) of pattern-reversal (check pattern counterphased at 1 Hz) and motion-onset (check pattern drifting at 6 deg/s) visually evoked potentials (VEPs), plotted as a function of Snellen acuity. Normal-eye data are plotted as open circles; amblyopic-eye data are plotted as solid circles. The amplitude and latency of the pattern-reversal VEP changed significantly (P < 0.001) with decreasing acuity (reprinted with permission from Kubova et al., 1996).*

that cortical areas served by the M pathway may be relatively spared in amblyopia.

MEG

The stimuli used in our MEG studies were photometrically isoluminant, red/green gratings (Anderson *et al.*, 1999). We chose this stimulus because the P pathway, which has an undisputed role in processing colour, may be more affected than the M pathway in amblyopia (e.g. Kubova *et al.*, 1996; Horton and Hocking, 1997); and because chromatic stimuli evoke strong magnetic responses from the occipital cortex of adults (Regan and He, 1996; Fylan *et al.*, 1997; Holliday *et al.*, 1997). The stimuli were approximately 5 degrees square, confined to a single visual quadrant for each set of measures. This was done in order to simplify the data analysis used in determining the site of cortical activity (see following section). Monocular evoked responses were recorded in a magnetically shielded room using a 19-channel MEG system (Matlashov *et al.*, 1995). Measures were completed on six strabismic adults and six normally-sighted adults. For all measures, the magnetometer was

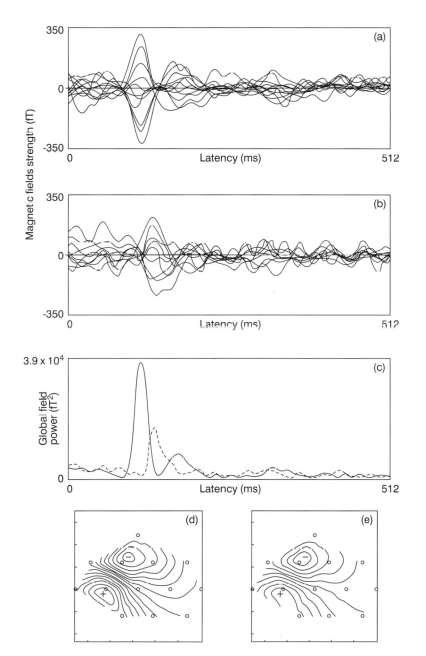

Figure 3.5 *MEG responses to the abrupt onset of a red/green sinusoid of 2 c/deg periodicity, positioned in the lower right visual field of amblyopic observer JD. Magnetic field strength for the normal (a) and amblyopic (b) eye plotted as a function of time from stimulus onset for each magnetometer channel. (c) The global evoked magnetic field power G(t) for the normal (solid line) and amblyopia eye (broken line), defined as:*

$$G(t) = \sum_{i=1}^{n} (A_i(t))^2$$

where $A_i(t)$ is the amplitude (fT) of the evoked magnetic signal in channel i at time t, and n is the number of operative channels. (d, e) Interpolated maps of magnetic field strength calculated at a latency corresponding to the peak in G(t) for the normal (d) and amblyopic (e) eye (reprinted with permission from Anderson et al., 1999).

centred on the midline of the subject's head, immediately above electrode position *Oz*.

Figure 3.5 shows, for both the (a) normal and (b) amblyopic eyes of subject JD, the amplitude of the evoked magnetic field plotted as a function of time from stimulus onset for each magnetometer channel. Note that, in comparison with the responses evoked by normal-eye stimulation, those evoked by amblyopic-eye stimulation were both delayed and reduced in amplitude. The global field power plots in panel (c) show this more clearly: field power peaked at 114 ms for the normal eye (solid line) and 137 ms for the amblyopic eye (broken line). The interpolated field profiles of magnetic field strength calculated at the time of the peak for each eye were similar: they each had a characteristic dipolar appearance consistent with neural activity arising from within a small region of cortex – panels (d) and (e).

Figure 3.6 shows global field power plots for the normal and amblyopic eyes of six subjects. The solid arrows point to the peak of the amblyopic functions. There were large individual differences in the maximum field power, the level of noise and the complexity of the function. However, the results for all six amblyopes were similar in that:

1. The responses for each eye were dominated by a single major peak in field power

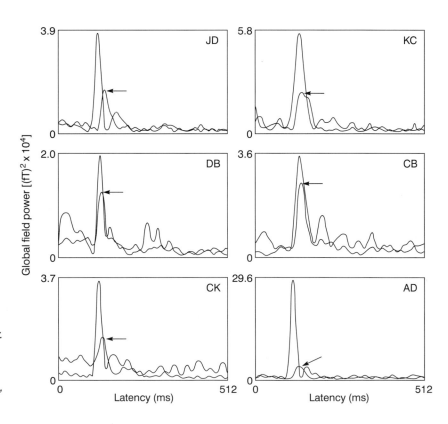

Figure 3.6 *Global field power plots for six strabismic amblyopes. In each case, the stimulus was a red/green sinusoid of 1–2 c/deg periodicity. The arrow in each panel points to the peak of the amblyopia-eye function (reprinted with permission from Anderson et al., 1999).*

2. The maximum power was always least with stimulation of the subject's amblyopic eye
3. The latency of this peak was always greatest with amblyopic-eye stimulation.

The interocular differences in latency (mean: 14 ms) and power (mean: 6×10^4 fT^2) were significant (Wilcoxon T = 0, two-tailed, $P < 0.05$).

Global field power plots, similar to those shown in Figure 3.6, were calculated for a range of stimulus periodicities. By plotting the maximum field power as a function of stimulus periodicity, we derived a measure of the spatial frequency response properties of the activated cortical area. Figure 3.7 shows the results for six amblyopes. The tuning functions for the normal (closed symbols) and amblyopic eyes (open symbols) of each subject were bandpass, peaking at 1–2 c/deg with a cut-off near 4 c/deg. Note that the

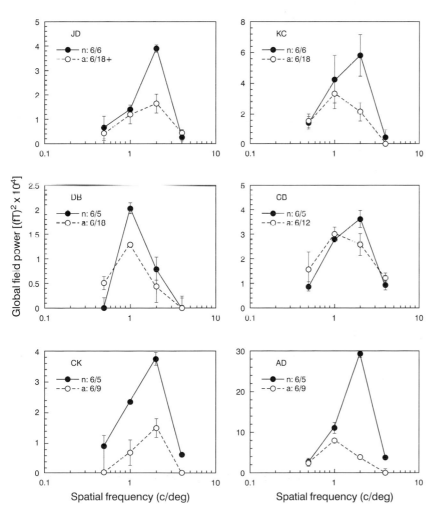

Figure 3.7 *The maximum value of G(t) (defined in Figure legend 3.5) for both normal- (solid circles) and amblyopia-eye (open circles) viewing plotted as a function of stimulus periodicity for six observers. Zero values of G(t) indicate that no major component was evident in the evoked response (reprinted with permission from Anderson et al., 1999).*

strength of the field power at the peak was significantly reduced through the amblyopic eye. Unlike Kubova and co-workers (1996), however, we did not find a good correlation between the amplitude of the responses driven by the amblyopic eye and monocular acuity. Barnes and co-workers (2001) also reported that the fMRI response reduction in amblyopia does not seem to relate to the subject's acuity deficit.

All of the above MEG measures and calculations were repeated for a control group of six normally-sighted adults. While statistical evaluation of the amblyopic group data showed that the magnetic evoked responses had significantly longer latencies and reduced power through the amblyopic eye ($P < 0.05$), evaluation of the control group revealed no significant interocular differences (Anderson *et al.*, 1999). These authors concluded that MEG is sensitive to the cortical deficit in strabismic amblyopia, and that the decreased magnetic response from the amblyopic eye of each subject can be attributed to dysfunction within their occipital cortex. The following section outlines how the site of dysfunction within the occipital cortex can be calculated from the recorded MEG signals.

NEURAL SITE OF AMBLYOPIC MEG RESPONSES

Figure 3.8 shows schematically the measured pattern of magnetic field strength evoked by our chromatic stimulus: the interpolated field profile is

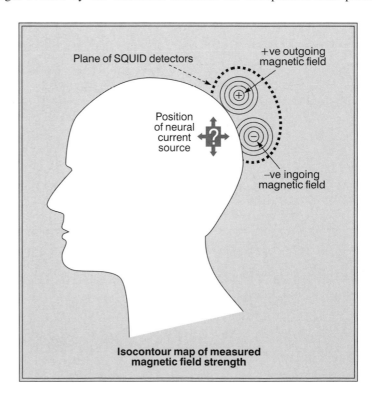

Figure 3.8 *Pictorial demonstration of* The Inverse Problem. *The interpolated isocontour map of magnetic field strength associated with evoked cortical activity lies in the plane of the SQUID detectors. The +ve and −ve regions of the map indicate the direction of the magnetic field. The problem is to determine the site (or sites) of cortical activity that gave rise to this particular magnetic field distribution at this particular spatial location above the patient's head.*

shown immediately above the observer's head in the plane occupied by the SQUID sensors. The task is to determine the site (or sites) of electrical activity in the observer's brain that gave rise to this particular magnetic field distribution at this particular location above the observer's head. This is termed 'the inverse problem'.

It is often stated that the inverse problem is insoluble (i.e. an infinite variety of current sources could give rise to the measured pattern of magnetic field strength). However, this is only true in the absence of any assumptions about the form of the neural current sources and conductive media. A common approach to solving this problem is to assume that the head is a uniform volume conductor with spherical symmetry, and that at any instant in time the neural currents can be represented as though they were produced by a single-equivalent current dipole. In essence, the inversion procedure reduces to finding the number and position of these dipoles. Best-fit solutions are usually determined using a non-linear, least-squares minimization procedure, taking into account the position and configuration of the SQUID detectors. Figure 3.9 shows a flow diagram summarizing the magnetic inversion procedure.

We have found in our experiments on amblyopes that a simple dipole model of the type described above can account for at least 97 per cent of the variance in the data (Anderson *et al.*, 1999). For each observer, there was no significant

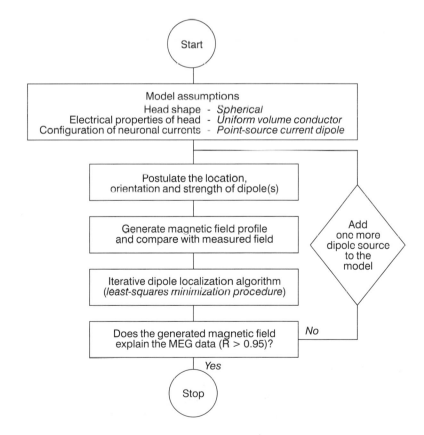

Figure 3.9 *Flow chart of the magnetic inversion procedure.*

Figure 3.10 *Monte Carlo generated ensemble of single equivalent current dipole source solutions to the visually evoked responses obtained from strabismic amblyope JD (raw data shown in Figure 3.5). This analysis was completed for a latency corresponding to the maximum evoked magnetic field power for JD, namely 114 ms for the normal eye and 137 ms for the amblyopic eye (see Figure 3.5c). The dipole ensemble is shown in three orthogonal spatial planes: the open symbols (amblyopic left eye) are plotted relative to the mean of the closed symbols (normal right eye), which is centred on the origin (x_o, y_o, z_o). Only measurement noise errors were incorporated into the analyses, calculated as the anti-average. The ensemble of dipoles for the right and left eye are not spatially distinct (P > 0.05).*

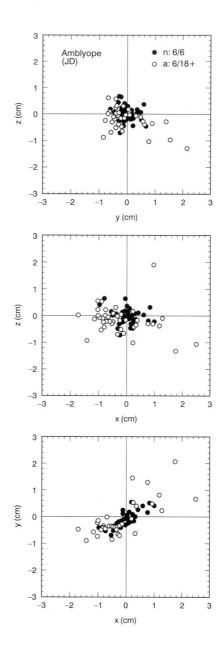

difference between the location of the right and left eye dipole fits, based on the 95 per cent confidence volume for the location of each dipole using a 40-trial Monte Carlo analysis (Singh *et al.*, 1997). The results of this procedure are shown in Figure 3.10 for one strabismic amblyope (JD), and in Figure 3.11 for one normally-sighted observer (IH). For each observer, dipole source analysis was applied at a latency corresponding to the peak in the major component of their magnetic field power functions (see Figure legends for details). Figures 3.10 and 3.11 show the generated dipoles in three

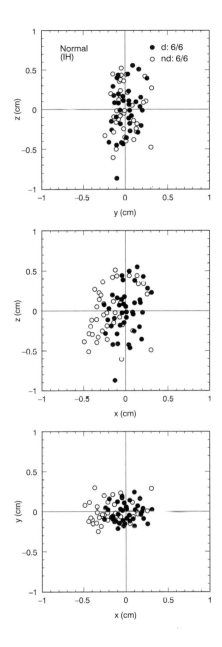

Figure 3.11 *As in Figure 3.10 for normally-sighted observer IH. The stimulus was a red/green sinusoid of 2 c/deg periodicity. The analysis was completed for a latency corresponding to the maximum evoked magnetic field power for IH, namely 136 ms for his dominant (right) eye and 137 ms for his non-dominant (left) eye. The ensemble of dipoles for the right and left eye were not spatially distinct (P > 0.05).*

orthogonal spatial planes, with the open symbols (left eye) plotted relative to the mean of the closed symbols (right eye), which was adjusted to zero in x, y, z space. For each eye of each observer, the centre of the dipole distributions was positioned near the midline beneath electrode position *Oz*, which is consistent with activity in area V1. Of note, we further determined that the location of the dipole source is not critically dependent on the latency at which the analysis is conducted. This is demonstrated in Figure 3.12, which shows, for observers JD and IH, the location of the right and left eye dipoles in x, y,

Figure 3.12 *Relative spatial location (in x, y, z space) of single dipole source solutions as a function of time from stimulus onset for a 15 ms span centred on the latency of the maximum evoked magnetic field power (indicated by vertical arrows) for normally-sighted observer IH and amblyopic observer JD. The source solutions are normalized with respect to their mean position (in x, y or z) for the 15 ms sample range. The single dipole model provided a good fit to the data at each position in time (R ≥ 0.99 for each eye of observer IH; R ≥ 0.97 for each eye of observer JD).*

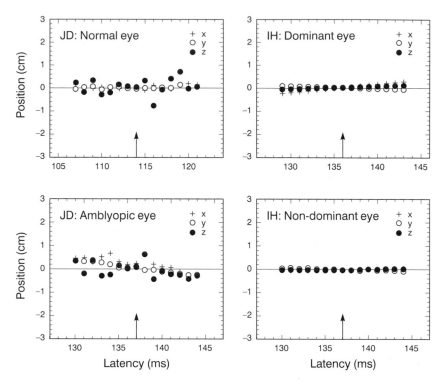

z space as a function of time from stimulus onset for a 15 ms span centred on the latency of the maximum evoked magnetic field power for each observer.

To estimate the site of neural activity more accurately, the dipole source solutions for observer IH were co-registered with his MRI data. Details of this co-registration procedure are given in Singh *et al.* (1997). Figure 3.13 shows the right and left eye solutions depicted as 95 per cent confidence ellipsoids on sagittal and horizontal MR images: the largest ellipsoid in each image is for the non-dominant eye. The centre of the confidence ellipsoid is located near the occipital pole, above the calcarine sulcus and to the left of the interhemispheric midline, consistent with stimulation near the fovea in the lower right visual field. Based on the conventions of Talairach and Tournoux's (1988) stereotaxic atlas, the activated cortical region is positioned at the junction of Brodmann's areas 17 and 18 (the Talairach co-ordinates for each eye are reported in the Figure legend). It has recently been reported, however, that the co-ordinates of Talairach and Tournoux's atlas tend to underestimate the extent of area 17 (Amunts *et al.*, 2000), in which case it may be that the activated neural region in our MEG experiments resides entirely within the striate cortex (V1). Nonetheless, based on our current results it is difficult to exclude the possibility that the extrastriate cortex (V2) was also activated. Perhaps this should not be too surprising given that, in monkeys at least, all submodalities of vision are represented in both areas (Shipp and Zeki, 1985).

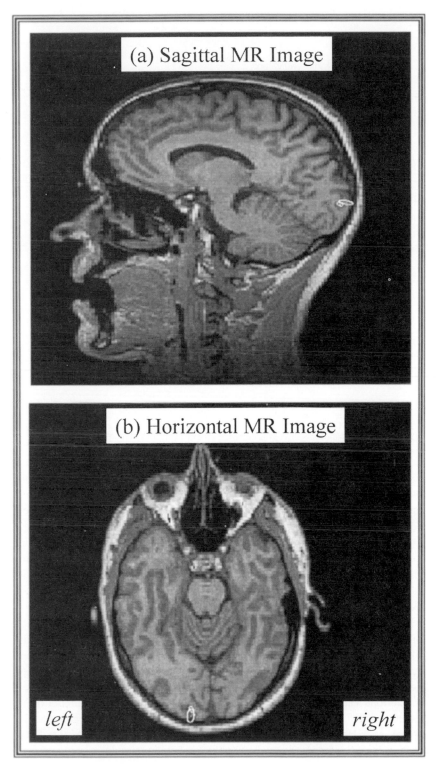

Figure 3.13 *Sagittal and horizontal MR images of normally-sighted observer IH co-registered with the 95 per cent confidence ellipsoids for the location of single dipole source solutions to responses evoked by a red/green sinusoid positioned in the lower, right visual field. The largest ellipsoid in each image is the solution for the non-dominant eye. The Talairach and Tournoux (1988) stereotaxic co-ordinates for the centre of each ellipsoid are: $x = -98$, $y = -10$, $z = +8$ for the dominant eye, and $x = -101$, $y = -10$, $z = +9$ for the non-dominant eye. These co-ordinates correspond to the junction of Brodmann's areas 17 and 18 (see Figure 117 of Talairach and Tournoux, 1988) (adapted with permission from Anderson et al., 1999).*

Figure 3.14 *Pictorial demonstration of the retinotopic organization of the primary visual cortex, area V1, here depicted according to the cruciform model of Jeffreys and Axford (1972). In the example shown, a stimulus positioned in the lower right visual field evokes activity above the calcarine sulcus and to the left of the interhemispheric midline. First-order modelling of the evoked activity by a current dipole source localizes the 'centre of mass' of the activated region. The direction of the dipole is given by the vector sum of the cortical currents.*

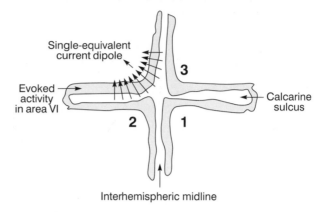

Cruciform model of primary visual cortex (VI)

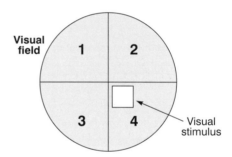

A further test of cortical activity within area V1 can be made by examining the change in dipole orientation as the stimulus is moved about the visual field. The architecture of V1 can be modelled as a cruciform because, despite intersubject variability in cortical anatomy, the calcarine sulcus (CS) and interhemispheric midline (IHM) tend to form a cross at the occipital pole (Jeffreys and Axford, 1972). Assuming this is the case, one should see a 90-degree change in dipole orientation as the stimulus is moved from one quadrant of the visual field to another. Figure 3.14 shows, for example, that a stimulus confined to the lower right visual field will evoke activity above CS and to the left of the IHM. This can be modelled as a single dipole source, the orientation of which is given by the vector sum of the neural currents.

Figure 3.15 shows, for one normally-sighted observer, maps of magnetic field strength for chromatic stimulation of each quadrant of the visual field – (a) upper left; (b) upper right; (c) lower left; (d) lower right. Each map was centred on or near electrode position *Oz* (Fylan *et al.*, 1997). For each map, the small arrow indicates the orientation of the dipole fit. Note that the dipole orientations vary in a way that is consistent with the cruciform model of V1 (Figure 3.14). These results, in conjunction with work by Regan and He (1996) and Holliday *et al.* (1997), led us to believe that a significant proportion of the responses evoked by our chromatic stimulus originated from

Maps of magnetic field strength

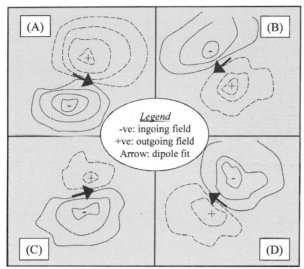

Figure 3.15 *Interpolated maps of magnetic field strength evoked by a red/green sinusoid positioned in each quadrant of the visual field – (a) upper left; (b) upper right; (c) lower left; (d) lower right. Each map was centred on or near electrode position Oz. The dipole source solution is shown as a small arrow in each map. See text for explanation (adapted with permission from Fylan et al., 1997).*

Stimulus location in visual field

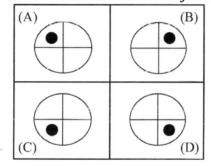

area V1. Therefore, the poor MEG responses obtained with stimulation of the amblyopic eye of our subjects presumably reflects cortical dysfunction within area V1.

CONCLUSIONS

Our MEG studies lead us to conclude that the poor spatial vision of amblyopes can, at least in part, be attributed to cortical dysfunction within area V1. This is in agreement with the large body of animal work that has been completed, and it also agrees with the recent fMRI work of Barnes *et al.* (1999, 2001). However, this conclusion runs contrary to the PET work of Imamura *et al.* (1997) and the fMRI work of Sireteanu *et al.* (1998).

What, if anything, do these disparate results tell us about the neural basis of amblyopia? The nature of the cortical deficit in amblyopia remains controversial although various proposals have been advanced, including neural disarray (e.g. Hess and Field, 1994), neural under-sampling (e.g. Levi and Klein, 1986), a loss of fine-scale spatial visual processing (Levi *et al.*, 1994), and desynchronized cortical responses (Roelfsema *et al.*, 1994). The synchronization model has received considerable attention lately. It is based on multi-electrode recordings from the striate cortex of strabismic cats, which indicate that the neuronal responses driven by the normal eye are more highly synchronized than those driven by the amblyopic eye.

None of these models alone can account for *all* the animal and human data, although together they can. The simplest explanation for this is that strabismic amblyopia may be associated with a variety of cortical deficits, not all of which are necessarily present in each individual. The nature of the deficit may depend on the type and degree of strabismus, whether or not it occurs in conjunction with a refractive error, and the age at which any treatment (patching and/or surgery) had been administered. A variety of cortical deficits have been found in primates with experimentally induced strabismus, although interestingly the nature of the physiological deficits appears more related to the depth of amblyopia than the type of amblyopia (Kiorpes *et al.*, 1998). To achieve consistent results, therefore, it may be necessary to secure a group of patients with the same depth of amblyopia.

A diverse subject pool could be one reason why Sireteanu *et al.* (1998) and Barnes *et al.* (1999, 2001) obtained different results despite using a similar fMRI-based experimental paradigm. Sireteanu and co-workers examined amblyopic subjects whose right and left eye acuity thresholds, assessed psychophysically using grating stimuli, differed by as little as one octave. These moderate amblyopes were found to have normal levels of cortical activity in area V1. On the other hand, Barnes and co-workers examined severe amblyopes and reported that V1 activity is abnormal. Therefore, fMRI may be insensitive to the cortical changes in V1 associated with mild to moderate amblyopia. Whether that is the case or not, the current disagreement between the fMRI studies needs to be resolved. In the absence of Barnes *et al.*'s data, Anderson *et al.* (1999) concluded that the most recent MEG, PET and fMRI data could be explained using the synchronization model of Roelfsema *et al.* (1994). As the amplitude of the extracranial evoked magnetic field increases with increasing synchronicity of the underlying neural population, Anderson *et al.* argued that the reduced MEG responses recorded in amblyopia may reflect desynchronized cortical activity (see also Roelfsema *et al.*, 1994). On the other hand, normal V1 activity might be expected using PET (Imamura *et al.*, 1997) and fMRI (Sireteanu *et al.*, 1998) because the poor temporal resolution of these techniques renders them insensitive to asynchronous firing on a millisecond time scale. Accepting the recent work of Barnes and co-workers, however, this conclusion is no longer tenable – at least not for severe amblyopes. This is not to discount asynchronous firing as a possible basis of amblyopia, but it does seem unlikely that it is the only neural correlate.

In summary, while agreement between neuroimaging studies is always welcome, discrepancies between them may be helpful in determining the neural basis of various visual disorders, including amblyopia. In this respect, the combined use of fMRI and MEG should be beneficial. At this stage, however, the basis of amblyopia remains a controversial issue, one which neuroimaging studies have yet to shed much light on. What does seem clear is that area V1 is the earliest site of dysfunction within the amblyopic visual system of humans. Both MEG and fMRI are sensitive to the deficits in this area, although they might not be apparent with fMRI unless the depth of amblyopia is severe. It is also clear from neuroimaging studies that there must be additional cortical deficits associated with amblyopia within visual areas beyond V1. This is important, because quantitative analyses have shown that the physiological deficits in V1 are not sufficient to explain the full range of perceptual deficits in amblyopia (Kiorpes *et al.*, 1998; Kiorpes and McKee, 1999).

ACKNOWLEDGEMENTS

The MEG work reported in this chapter was supported by Fight For Sight, London. Parts of this chapter were written while on leave at ATR Human Information Processing Research Laboratories in Kyoto, Japan. I thank all the members in Department 5 at ATR for their support, especially Dr Noriko Yamagishi. I also thank Drs Gareth Barnes, Arjan Hillebrand and Ian Holliday for several useful discussions, and for reading draft sections of this chapter.

REFERENCES

Aine, C. J. (1995). A conceptual overview and critique of functional neuroimaging techniques in humans: I. MRI/fMRI and PET. *Crit. Rev. Neurobiol.*, **9**, 229–309.

Aine, C. J., Supek, S., George, J. *et al.* (1995). MEG studies of human vision: retinotopic organization of V1. In: *Biomagnetism: Fundamental Research and Clinical Applications* (C. Baumgartner, L. Deecke, G. Stroink *et al.*, eds.), pp. 153–61. Elsevier Science, IOS Press.

Anderson, S. J. and Holliday, I. E. (1998). Assessment of cortical dysfunction in human amblyopia using magneto-encephalography (MEG). *Inv. Ophthalmol. Vis. Sci.*, **39**, S909.

Anderson, S. J., Holliday, I. E., Singh, K. D. and Harding, G. F. A. (1996). Localization and functional analysis of human cortical area V5 using magneto-encephalography. *Proc. R. Soc. Lond. Series B*, **263**, 423–31.

Anderson, S. J., Holliday, I. E. and Harding, G. F. A. (1999). Assessment of cortical dysfunction in human strabismic amblyopia using magneto-encephalography (MEG). *Vision Res.*, **39**, 1723–38.

Amunts, K., Malikovic, A., Mohlberg, H. *et al.* (2000). Brodmann's areas 17 and 18 brought into stereotaxic space – where and how variable. *NeuroImage*, **11**, 66–84.

Barnes, G. R., Hess, R. F., Petre, V. *et al.* (1999). FMRI responses to sinusoidal grating stimuli in strabismic amblyopes. *Inv. Ophthalmol. Vis. Sci.*, **40**, S644.

Barnes, G. R., Hess, R. F., Dumoulin, S. O. *et al.* (2001). The cortical deficit in humans with strabismic amblyopia. *J. Physiol.*, **533**, 281–97.

Blakemore, C. (1990). Maturation of mechanisms for efficient spatial vision. In: *Vision: Coding and Efficiency* (C. Blakemore, ed.), pp. 254–66. Cambridge University Press.

Crewther, D. P. and Crewther, S. G. (1990). Neural site of strabismic amblyopia in cats: spatial frequency deficit in primary cortical neurons. *Exp. Brain Res.*, **79**, 615–22.

Demer, J. L. (1993). Positron emission tomographic studies of cortical function in human amblyopia. *Neurosci. Biobehav. Rev.*, **17**, 469–76.

Demer, J. L., Noorden, G. K., Volkow, N. D. and Gould, K. L. (1988). Imaging of cerebral blood flow and metabolism in amblyopia by positron emission tomography. *Am. J. Ophthalmol.*, **105**, 337–47.

Fylan, F., Holliday, I. E., Singh, K. D. *et al.* (1997). Magneto-encephalographic investigation of human cortical area V1 using color stimuli. *NeuroImage*, **6**, 47–57.

Hajnal, J. V., Myers, R., Oatridge, A. *et al.* (1994). Artifacts due to stimulus correlated motion in functional imaging of the brain. *Mag. Res. Med.*, **31**, 283–91.

Hämäläinen, M., Hari, R., Ilmoniemi, R. J. *et al.* (1993). Magneto-encephalography – theory, instrumentation, and applications to non-invasive studies of the working human brain. *Rev. Mod. Physics*, **65**, 413–97.

Hartshorne, M. F. (1995). Positron emission tomography. In: *Functional Brain Imaging* (W. W. Orrison, J. D. Lewine, J. A. Sanders and M. F. Hartshorne, eds), pp. 187–212. Mosby Year Book, Inc.

Hess, R. F. and Field, D. J. (1994). Is the spatial deficit in strabismic amblyopia due to loss of cells or an uncalibrated disarray of cells? *Vision Res.*, **34**, 3397–406.

Hess, R. F., Field, D. J. and Watt, R. J. (1990). The puzzle of amblyopia. In: *Vision: Coding and Efficiency* (C. Blakemore, ed.), pp. 267–80. Cambridge University Press.

Hillebrand, A. (2000). The development of constrained source localization algorithms for human brain imaging. PhD thesis, Aston University.

Holliday, I. E., Anderson, S. J. and Harding, G. F. A. (1997). Magneto-encephalographic evidence for non-geniculostriate visual input to human cortical area V5. *Neuropsychologia*, **35**, 1139–46.

Horton, J. C. and Hocking, D. R. (1996). Pattern of ocular dominance columns in human striate cortex in strabismic amblyopia. *Vis. Neurosci.*, **13**, 787–95.

Horton, J. C. and Hocking, D. R. (1997). Timing of the critical period for plasticity of ocular dominance columns in macaque striate cortex. *J. Neurosci.*, **17**, 3684–709.

Horton, J. C. and Stryker, M. P. (1993). Amblyopia induced by anisometropia without shrinkage of ocular dominance columns in human striate cortex. *Proc. Natl Acad. Sci. USA*, **90**, 5494–8.

Imamura, K., Richter, H., Fischer, H. *et al.* (1997). Reduced activity in the extrastriate visual cortex of individuals with strabismic amblyopia. *Neurosci. Lett.*, **225**, 173–6.

Jeffreys, D. A. and Axford, J. G. (1972). Source locations of pattern specific components of human visual evoked potentials. I. Components of striate cortical origin. *Exp. Brain Res.*, **16**, 1–21.

Kiorpes, L. and McKee, S. P. (1999). Neural mechanisms underlying amblyopia. *Curr. Opin. Neurobiol.*, **9**, 480–86.

Kiorpes, L., Kiper, D. C., O'Keefe, L. P. *et al.* (1998). Neuronal correlates of amblyopia in the visual cortex of macaque monkeys with experimental strabismus and anisometropia. *J. Neurosci.*, **18**, 6411–24.

Kubova, Z., Kuba, M., Juran, J. and Blakemore, C. (1996). Is the motion system relatively spared in amblyopia? Evidence from cortical evoked responses. *Vision Res.*, **36**, 181–90.

Le Goualher, G., Procyk, E., Collins, D. L. *et al.* (1999). Automated extraction and variabilty analysis of sulcal neuroanatomy. *IEEE Trans. Medical Imaging*, **18**, 206–17.

Levi, D. M. and Klein, S. A. (1986). Sampling in spatial vision. *Nature (Lond.)*, **320**, 360–62.

Levi, D. M., Waugh, S. J. and Beard, B. L. (1994). Spatial scale shifts in amblyopia. *Vision Res.*, **34**, 3315–33.

Lewine, J. D. and Orrison, W. W. (1995). Magneto-encephalography and magnetic source imaging. In: *Functional Brain Imaging* (W. W. Orrison, J. D. Lewine, J. A. Sanders and M. F. Hartshorne, eds), pp. 369–417. Mosby Year Book, Inc.

Logothetis, N. K., Pauls, J., Augath, M. *et al.* (2001). Neurophysiological investigation of the basis of the fMRI signal. *Nature (Lond.)*, **412**, 150–57.

Martin, G.N. (1998). *Human Neuropsychology*. Prentice Hall Europe.

Matlashov, A., Slobodchikov, V., Bakharev, A. *et al.* (1995). Biomagnetic multichannel system built with 19 cryogenic probes. In: *Biomagnetism: Fundamental Research and Clinical*

Applications (C. Baumgartner, L. Deeke, G. Sroink and S. J. Williamson, eds), pp. 493–6. Elsevier Science, IOS Press.

Movshon, J. A. and Kiorpes, L. (1990). The role of experience in visual development. In: *Development of Sensory Systems in Mammals* (J. R. Coleman, ed.), pp. 155–202. Wiley.

Ogawa, S., Lee, L. M., Kay, A. R. and Tank, D. W. (1990). Brain magnetic resonance imaging with contrast dependent on blood oxygenation. *Proc. Natl Acad. Sci.*, **87**, 9868–72.

Orrison, W. W., Lewine, J. D., Sanders, J. A. and Hartshorne, M. F. (1995). *Functional Brain Imaging*. Mosby.

Regan, D. (1989). *Human Brain Electrophysiology – Evoked Potentials and Evoked Magnetic Fields in Science and Medicine*. Elsevier Science.

Regan, D. and He, P. (1996). Magnetic and electrical brain responses to chromatic contrast in human. *Vision Res.*, **36**, 1 18.

Roelfsema, P. R., Konig, P., Engel, A. K. *et al.* (1994). Reduced synchronization in the visual cortex of cats with strabismic amblyopia. *Eur. J. Neurosci.*, **6**, 1645–55.

Romani, G. L., Williamson, S. J. and Kaufman, L. (1982). Biomagnetic instrumentation. *Rev. Scient. Instrument.*, **53**, 1815–45.

Shipp, S. and Zeki, S. M. (1985) Segregation of pathways leading from area V2 to areas V4 and V5 of macaque visual cortex. *Nature (Lond.)*, **315**, 322–5.

Singh, K. D., Holliday, I. E., Furlong, P. L. and Harding, G. F. A. (1997). Evaluation of MRI–MEG/EEG co-registration strategies using Monte Carlo simulation. *Electrophysiol. Clin. Neurophysiol.*, **102**, 81–5.

Sireteanu, R., Tonhausen, N., Muckli, L. *et al.* (1998). Cortical site of the amblyopic deficit in strabismic and anisometropic subjects investigated with fMRI. *Inv. Ophthalmol. Vis. Sci.*, **39**, S909.

Talairach, J. and Tournoux, P. (1988) *Co-planar Stereotaxic Atlas of the Human Brain*. Thieme.

Toga, A. W. and Mazziotta, J. C. (1996). *Brain Mapping*. Academic Press.

Tootell, R. B. H., Reppas, J. B., Kwong, K. K. *et al.* (1995). Functional analysis of human MT and related visual cortical areas using magnetic-resonance-imaging. *J. Neurosci.*, **15**, 3215–30.

Van Essen, D. C. and Drury, H. A. (1997). Structural and functional analyses of human cerebral cortex using a surfaced-based atlas. *J. Neurosci.*, **17**, 7079–102.

Van Essen, D. C., Maunsell, J. H. R. and Bixby, J. L. (1981). The middle temporal area in the macaque: myeloarchitecture, connections, functional properties and topographic organisation. *J. Comp. Neurol.*, **199**, 293–326.

Zeki, S. M. (1974). Functional organisation of a visual area in the posterior bank of the superior temporal sulcusin the rhesus monkey. *J. Physiol. Lond.*, **236**, 549–73.

Zeki, S. M., Watson, J. D. G., Lueck, C. J. *et al.* (1991). A direct demonstration of functional specialization in human visual cortex. *J. Neurosc.*, **11**, 641–9.

4 Taxonomy and epidemiology of amblyopia

Barnaby C. Reeves

INTRODUCTION

This chapter considers amblyopia in the applied context of health services research and health technology assessment (see NHS Management Executive, 1992). It therefore offers a different perspective from most of the other contributions in this monograph, whose predominant concerns are the neuroscientific and clinical aspects of the condition.

From the standpoint of health services, amblyopia can be a frustrating subject to study. My aim here is to try to highlight some of the reasons for these frustrations. I shall review some of what we know about the epidemiology of amblyopia, primarily from a descriptive rather than an aetiological point of view. A systematic review (e.g. see Chalmers *et al.*, 1989; Chalmers and Altman, 1995) is not attempted, and I accept the criticism that I have chosen examples to make particular points. However, I believe that the advantages of a systematic approach are not essential for my thesis – namely that we are somewhat ignorant with regard to the basic epidemiology of amblyopia and that our lack of knowledge has implications for treatment evaluation.

The chapter tackles four issues. First, I will examine critically the definitions of amblyopia used previously by researchers to illustrate practical problems that they raise for researchers. Second, I will describe taxonomies of amblyopia that have been proposed and question their robustness. Third, I will review epidemiological evidence about the validity or usefulness of a taxonomy, i.e. the extent to which it helps to explain the diversity of functional loss and visual outcome that has been observed clinically. Fourth, I consider the implications of gaps in our knowledge for evaluations of treatments for amblyopia.

DEFINITIONS OF AMBLYOPIA

Von Noorden (1985) provided a widely accepted clinical definition of amblyopia:

> A unilateral or bilateral decrease of visual acuity caused by form vision deprivation and/or abnormal binocular interaction for which no organic causes can be detected by the physical examination of the eye and which, in appropriate cases, is reversible by therapeutic measures.

This definition has certain features. First, it is an operational or functional definition, starting as it does with the clinical observation of 'a unilateral or bilateral decrease of visual acuity . . .'. Second, it is a definition by exclusion – that is, a diagnosis of amblyopia should only be assigned when '. . . no organic {ocular} causes can be detected . . .'. Finally, the definition includes reference to prognosis – that is, amblyopic visual loss '. . . in appropriate cases is reversible by therapeutic measures'. Variations on this definition have been formulated, but they retain the majority of these features (Ciuffreda et al., 1991).

Definitions of this kind are not uncommon in medicine, and they are usually sufficiently precise for clinical purposes. I am not criticizing the principle of formulating a definition in this way, but do want to point out that such a definition can be difficult to apply consistently in a research context, since operational criteria:

- may be set at different 'thresholds' across studies
- may be difficult to measure or ascertain
- may be susceptible to bias
- are often applied in a pragmatic fashion.

Measurements of visual acuity serve to illustrate the first three points. With respect to the threshold problem, at what level of visual acuity should a child be considered to have a ' . . . decrease in visual acuity . . .'? In terms of ascertainment, should it be a requirement that the decrease in visual acuity observed on one occasion be seen on a second occasion, or some similar criterion to reduce misclassification, given the variability in measurement of children's visual acuity (Kheterpal et al., 1996)? How should one accommodate different visual acuity tests, or children who prove difficult to test? It is no surprise that measures made in these circumstances can be susceptible to biases unless great care is taken to avoid them, for example by masking the person carrying out the assessment. These measures are unlikely to occur in normal health care practice, and even in a research setting it is important to test whether or not masking has been successful (Begg et al., 1996).

Of course, these problems do not only affect visual acuity measurements. Ocular movements and other clinical signs important in the classification of amblyopia are similarly difficult to measure. Assessment of both visual acuity and ocular movements is complicated by the presence of refractive error, measurement of which is also variable.

Operational criteria for amblyopia are also susceptible to bias because of the complex way in which clinical signs influence the decision to assign the diagnosis. Amblyopia is not, in fact, diagnosed simply by exclusion of an 'organic cause', but is also influenced by the presence of other signs, such as strabismus, phoria and anisometropia. In practice, a clinician constantly revises the probability of a child having amblyopia, taking into account all the other information that is available. Most of the other relevant clinical signs are also defined operationally and are difficult to measure. As a clinician's index of suspicion varies, so too may the rigour with which he or she looks for signs in the absence of an unexplained visual acuity deficit.

Variation in the application of a definition poses serious problems for scientific investigation. The situation is often exacerbated by the failure of authors to provide details of the operational criteria adopted and the methods of measurement. Thus there is plenty of scope for variation between studies that is not just due to chance or 'real' differences, making it difficult to know exactly who has been included and excluded.

The difficulty in making a definitive diagnosis of amblyopia has led to a tendency amongst researchers to classify vision problems in children in terms of observable signs (Stayte *et al.*, 1990, 1993). The need for longitudinal information to confirm a diagnosis of amblyopia may also help to explain this phenomenon, although this should not be a problem in retrospective studies. The alternative, pragmatic approach, is simply to classify children as having amblyopia if they are treated for it, i.e. receive occlusion therapy (Woodruff *et al.*, 1994a, 1994b; Reeves and Stayte, unpublished observations). Clearly, this approach merely disguises the issues that a clinician has to weigh up, as discussed above, in coming to a decision to begin treatment.

In summary:

1. A definition of amblyopia is difficult to apply consistently
2. Inconsistent application of a definition makes it difficult to compare findings from one study to another without detailed specification of the definitions adopted and other details, for example about the methods of measurement of visual performance and clinical signs
3. Inconsistent application of a definition makes it difficult to attribute discrepant findings in the literature to, for example, differences in clinical populations, bias or chance.

TAXONOMY OF AMBLYOPIA

Ideally, a classification system for amblyopia should explain some of the variation observed between amblyopic patients by, for example, defining subcategories of amblyopia with differing aetiology, severity of disease or variation in prognosis. Identifying types of amblyopia with differing prognosis would be of particular interest, given the wide variation in outcome that has been documented amongst amblyopic patients. The extent of the variation in outcome has been described in a number of studies (Ingram *et al.*, 1986; Lithander and Sjöstrand, 1991; Hiscox *et al.*, 1992; Reeves and Stayte, unpublished observations), and can range from no improvement up to six lines or more on a letter acuity chart.

Von Noorden (1985) distinguished between abnormal binocular interaction (active inhibition of foveal vision in the affected eye to eliminate sensory interference) and deprivation of form vision as causes of different clinically

Table 4.1 Putative mechanisms underlying amblyopia (von Noorden, 1985)

Putative cause of amblyopia	Abnormal binocular interaction	Deprivation of form vision
Strabismus	Yes	No
Anisometropia	Yes	Yes
Visual deprivation:		
unilateral	Yes	Yes
bilateral	No	Yes

observed types of amblyopia, i.e. strabismic amblyopia, anisometropic amblyopia and amblyopia resulting from visual deprivation (see Table 4.1). Ciuffreda *et al.* (1991) make a further distinction within strabismic amblyopia between diplopia and confusion, the former arising because the image of the fixated object falls on non-corresponding retinal points in the two eyes and the latter arising because dissimilar objects are imaged on the foveas of the two eyes. However, the authors do not elaborate the importance of this distinction, hypothesizing that both problems lead to suppression.

Although von Noorden (1985) suspected that most anisometropes have microstrabismus, he argued that anisometropes experienced abnormal binocular interaction because of superimposition of a focused and unfocused image, and not because of a micro-deviation. He cited the observation that anisometropic amblyopia is more common and more severe in hypermetropes than myopes as evidence of the separate actions of the two mechanisms, with the affected eyes of hypermetropes but not myopes being subject to visual deprivation. In further support of the model, von Noorden also stated that unilateral deprivation, in which both mechanisms are again implicated by the model, leads to more severe amblyopia than bilateral deprivation.

On the same principle, one might expect anisometropic amblyopia to be more severe than strabismic amblyopia, and to have a similar natural history and prognosis to unilateral deprivation amblyopia. However, recent studies have consistently found pure anisometropic amblyopia to be less severe than strabismic amblyopia, with 'mixed' amblyopia (where both strabismus and anisometropia are present) having the worst severity of all on presentation (Ingram *et al.*, 1986; Stayte *et al.*, 1993) and poorer prognosis after treatment (Lithander and Sjöstrand, 1991; Woodruff *et al.*, 1994a).

These results have led researchers to distinguish a category of 'mixed' aetiology, separate from pure strabismic amblyopia. Classification is further complicated by the presence of microstrabismus, commonly found with anisometropia. Of course, the problem of choosing and applying unambiguous definitions (see previous section) also applies to subtypes of amblyopia. For example, depending upon the refractive error threshold for classifying a child as anisometropic, the definition adopted by investigators for classifying microtropia and the care taken to detect microtropia, patients may be included in different categories.

Categorization of children with microtropia deserves special consideration. Most early studies of the prevalence of different kinds of amblyopia failed to measure fixation, and are therefore likely to have included amblyopic children with anisometropia and microtropia as anisometropic amblyopes (Ciuffreda *et al.*, 1991). The importance of children with anisometropia and microtropia in any taxonomy is illustrated by a study carried out by Flynn and Cassady (1978), in which 20 per cent of all amblyopes had this combination of visual defects. This proportion is much larger than the 6 per cent found in a retrospective review of all children referred for occlusion therapy (Woodruff *et al.*, 1994a), although this latter proportion may have underestimated the true proportion because of incomplete ascertainment of straight-eyed amblyopes (see below).

It is ironical, given the potential importance of these distinctions – especially the presence of microtropia (Helveston and von Noorden, 1967; von Noorden, 1985; Almeder *et al.*, 1990; Ciuffreda *et al.*, 1991) – that past studies have often failed to report these details unequivocally. It is not sufficient to assume that a category labelled 'anisometropic amblyopia' excludes children with a microtropia, since operational criteria for detecting a microtropia may vary, and microtropia may be explicitly included as part of the syndrome of anisometropic amblyopia (Helveston and von Noorden, 1967; Hardman Lea *et al.*, 1989). Recent longitudinal studies have also highlighted the importance of microtropia, and have raised interesting questions about the causal relationships between anisometropia, microtropia and amblyopia – for example, is microtropia the cause or the consequence of anisometropia (Almeder *et al.*, 1990; Abrahamsson and Sjostrand, 1996; Fielder and Moseley, 1996)? If the cause, then can anisometropic amblyopia develop in the absence of a microtropia (von Noorden, 1985)? If not, the aetiology, or natural history, of children presenting with 'pure anisometropia' needs clarification.

Almost all studies investigating outcome for different types of amblyopia have been retrospective, and therefore susceptible to bias and confounding. For example, in case note reviews it is difficult to mask classification of the type of amblyopia to knowledge about the treatment given or the outcome attained, making such studies susceptible to differential bias. One small prospective study (Lithander and Sjöstrand, 1991) found a contradictory result with respect to prognosis compared with the retrospective ones (Hiscox *et al.*, 1992; Woodruff *et al.*, 1994b). Lithander and Sjöstrand observed that there was no difference in the proportion of strabismic and anisometropic amblyopes who recovered good vision in the affected eye when they complied with treatment.

Associations between type of amblyopia and outcome are inevitably confounded by other suspected prognostic factors such as age at onset or time of presentation, since anisometropic amblyopes tend to present at an older age. Multivariate analyses, which attempt to disentangle the independent effects of type of amblyopia, age at presentation, intensity and duration of treatment, are rare (e.g. Woodruff *et al.*, 1994b).

In summary, there is no high quality evidence to indicate that either von Noorden's (1985) original taxonomy, or one that includes a mixed category and differentiates anisometropes with and without microstrabismus, is useful in explaining the wide variation in outcome that is commonly observed.

Children who appear to be 'straight-eyed' but who are at risk of developing amblyopia for some reason are particularly important with respect to decisions about health services, since these children can develop profound amblyopia unnoticed by parents or health care professionals. The above discussion highlights that there may be subcategories of amblyopia with different 'risk' factors, with potential relevance to aetiology and prognosis. These factors include (Schapero, 1971; Ciuffreda et al., 1991):

1. Spherical anisometropia
2. Spherical anisomyopia
3. Astigmatic anisometropia
4. Presence of microtropia
5. Presence of phoria.

A similar situation arises for strabismic amblyopia, although it has attracted less interest. Factors of potential importance with respect to aetiology and prognosis include (Schapero, 1971; Ciuffreda et al., 1991):

1. Direction of primary deviation, i.e. esotropia or exotropia
2. Magnitude of deviation
3. Constancy of strabismus
4. Presence of a vertical deviation
5. Presumed cause of the strabismus, e.g. congenital/accommodative/other.

EPIDEMIOLOGY OF AMBLYOPIA

Estimates of the prevalence or cumulative incidence of amblyopia vary between 1.6 and 3.5 per cent (see Table 4.2; also Ciuffreda et al., 1991). Such variation is perhaps not surprising, given the problems in defining amblyopia and associated clinical signs. However, there are other possible sources of variation that may contribute to the range of estimates observed, including:

● study design, e.g. population-based surveys (Thompson et al., 1991), follow-up of defined populations such as birth cohorts (Stayte et al., 1990, 1993) and reviews of referrals (Woodruff et al., 1994a, 1994b)
● measure of disease frequency, i.e. prevalence or incidence
● characteristics of study population, e.g. age when surveyed.

There is an association between study design and the measure of disease frequency described by a study. Population-based surveys are usually cross-sectional and estimate prevalence directly from a defined denominator and numerator, although varying levels of non-participation in the study may introduce bias. Studies that follow up a birth cohort usually estimate cumulative incidence by a certain age directly from a defined denominator

Table 4.2 Estimates of the prevalence and incidence of amblyopia

Reference	Study design	Study population	Amblyopia criterion	Measure of disease frequency and estimate
Köhler and Stigmar, 1973	Population survey	Children examined at 4 years	Visual acuity = 6/18 or worse	Prevalence at 4 years = 1.8%
Thompson et al., 1991	Retrospective review of referrals	All children referred during one year (1983)	Visual acuity = 6/12 or worse	Incidence = 3.0%
Abrahamsson et al., 1992	Follow-up of birth cohort	All children born during 1979–1980	Visual acuity = 6/12 or worse	Cumulative incidence by 6 years = 4.1%
Reeves and Stayte, unpublished observations	Follow-up of birth cohort	All children born in 1984 and referred before 8 years	Treated with occlusion therapy	Cumulative incidence by 5 years = 1.6%
Attebo et al., 1998	Population survey	Adults ≥ 49 years	Visual acuity = 6/12 or worse	Prevalence at > 49 years = 2.9%

and numerator, although the numerator is likely to be derived by reviewing referrals retrospectively on the assumption that all affected patients are referred. In practice, therefore, many such studies offer little advantage over estimates of cumulative evidence by a certain age derived from retrospective reviews of referrals, where the denominator can be inferred from routine data characterizing the catchment population for a referral centre, and the numerator is the total number of affected patients that are referred. The assumption that all affected patients are referred means that the latter two study designs are highly dependent on the infrastructure for detecting vision defects. They are unlikely to provide reliable findings unless effective population screening programmes are in place.

The age of the population is also a possible source of variation in the estimated disease frequency. Estimates of prevalence will only be the same as estimates of cumulative incidence if cases of amblyopia never resolve spontaneously and if successfully treated cases are included in the numerator; in practice, successfully treated or prevented cases of amblyopia may not be detected in surveys of adults (Ciuffreda et al., 1991).

The dependence of follow-up studies of birth cohorts and retrospective reviews of referrals on the infrastructure for detecting vision defects has an even more important effect on estimates of the proportion of amblyopia arising from different postulated causes, since strabismic or mixed amblyopia is more likely to be referred spontaneously than anisometropic or straight-eyed amblyopia (see Table 4.3). Woodruff et al. (1994a) estimated that pure anisometropic amblyopia accounted for 17 per cent of amblyopes referred for treatment. This percentage increased to 23 per cent after re-classifying

Table 4.3 Estimates of the proportion of cases of amblyopia classified as anisometropic, strabismic or mixed

Reference	Anisometropic amblyopia (%)	'Mixed' amblyopia (%)	Strabismic amblyopia (%)
Thompson et al., 1991	17	27[a]	56
Flynn and Cassady, 1978	20	32[a]	48
Abrahamsson et al., 1992	67	33[b]	
Attebo et al., 1998[c]	50	27	19

[a]Includes anisometropic amblyopes with microstrabismus
[b]Combined 'mixed' and strabismic amblyopia and assumed to include anisometropic amblyopes with microstrabismus
[c]An additional 4 per cent of amblyopes were classified as having been caused by visual deprivation.

children with microtropia (originally classified as having amblyopia of mixed aetiology) as anisometropic. The authors concluded that differences in the classification of children with microtropia could not explain the discrepancy with birth cohorts and population-based surveys (Abrahamsson et al., 1992; Attebo et al., 1998), which estimated that anisometropic amblyopia accounted for a much greater proportion (50–67 per cent) of all amblyopes. They also found considerable variation between referral centres in the proportion of amblyopes classified as anisometropic, and they concluded that failure of health systems to refer children with anisometropic amblyopia may be an important factor when interpreting epidemiological studies. The lack of precision about subgroup membership makes statistics such as these even more unreliable.

Varying criteria for classifying a child as anisometropic can also contribute to the variation in the proportion of children in different categories. The degree of anisometropia that is required to be amblyogenic differs for hypermetropia and myopia (Ciuffreda et al., 1991), a point not appreciated in studies that have simply adopted a global criterion, e.g. >1.0 dioptre difference between eyes, without consideration of the nature of the refractive error.

Studies have also described the proportions of patients with different postulated causes who become amblyopic. Estimates for the proportion of strabismic children who become amblyopic vary from 21 per cent of exotropes (Catford et al., 1984) and 53 per cent (Catford et al., 1984) to 70 per cent of esotropes (Köhler and Stigmar, 1973), with an estimate of 53 per cent for all children with manifest strabismus (including microtropia; Abrahamsson et al., 1992).

There are several reasons why some strabismic patients may not develop amblyopia, for example alternating fixation, an intermittent squint, age of onset, etc. Such factors may allow the variation in these figures to be reconciled. For example, Köhler and Stigmar (1973) studied younger children in whom the development of amblyopia was more likely – i.e. children who developed strabismus after 4 years of age and who may have been less likely to develop amblyopia could not have been identified.

The proportion of anisometropes developing amblyopia is of particular interest, in view of debate about the cause and effect role of microtropia. Almeder *et al.* (1990) suggested that no infants had persistent anisometropia over time, i.e. anisometropia decayed with time; Abrahamsson and Sjöstrand (1996) have also suggested that development of amblyopia/microtropia precedes development of anisometropia. If microtropia (or other factors) is the cause of anisometropia (and amblyopia), then 'anisometropic' amblyopia (perhaps a misnomer?) should only occur in the presence of other amblyogenic factors, e.g. microtropia. It does not appear, however, that all 'anisometropic' amblyopes have an observable microtropia.

It is also important to point out that it is difficult to estimate the proportion of anisometropes who become amblyopic, since such an estimate requires a longitudinal and population-based study. Without a population-based study one cannot be sure that all children with anisometropia have been identified, and without close longitudinal follow-up one cannot identify children who become amblyopic because of their anisometropia.

It seems intuitive to suppose that the probability of a child developing amblyopia should be related to the degree of anisometropia. Woodruff *et al.* (1994b) found support for this view in their retrospective review of the outcome of children treated for amblyopia. Although they did not relate presenting visual acuity to the degree of anisometropia, visual acuity after treatment was strongly related to the difference in spherical equivalent between eyes, both for pure anisometropic amblyopes and for mixed amblyopes.

IMPLICATIONS FOR EVALUATIONS OF TREATMENT

As already described, previous studies have demonstrated a wide range of outcome in children treated for amblyopia. The majority achieve a modest gain, with a median of one to two lines on a Snellen chart (Ingram *et al.*, 1986; Lithander and Sjöstrand, 1991; Woodruff *et al.*, 1994b). However, a minority of about 10 per cent show substantial improvements in visual acuity (Ingram *et al.*, 1986). Also, using different definitions, two of these studies showed very high rates of success of treatment; Lithander and Sjöstrand (1991) observed that over 95 per cent of children who complied well with treatment were successfully treated (difference between eyes less than or equal to one Snellen line), and Woodruff *et al.* (1994b) found that 83 per cent of children had a visual acuity outcome of 6/18 or better in the affected eye.

With the current emphasis on randomized controlled trials (RCTs) (Jaeschke and Sackett 1989; NHS Management Executive, 1992), it is easy to forget that there is a hierarchy of evidence of effectiveness (Elwood, 1998) and that it may not be necessary to evaluate a treatment using an RCT if the treatment has been demonstrated to have a large effect using study designs that are more susceptible to bias (Black, 1996). Indeed it might even be considered unethical to randomize patients to treatment or not, in the face of evidence of a large effect of a treatment from non-randomized studies.

Existing evidence about the size of the effect has been obtained mainly using uncontrolled before–after study designs; such studies are correctly viewed as being of poor quality in the hierarchy of evidence. Given that, typically, only a minority of patients achieve large gains in visual acuity, the overall effect of treatment for amblyopia is not large enough to exclude bias as a possible explanation of the findings. However, the effect of treatment amongst those who benefit the most certainly appears to be large, and it seems unlikely that such a large effect could arise from bias.

It may be the case that the outcome of treatment is completely independent of the treatment itself, and that some large improvements in a minority of patients are just part of the natural history of amblyopia. However, this seems quite a dangerous position to take in view of the established nature of occlusion treatment and the clear comparative evidence that exists of reversibility. Modest improvements may be just a practice or placebo effect, but it is difficult to explain large improvements in this way.

Another possibility is that there is heterogeneity amongst amblyopes with respect to outcome, i.e. there may be subgroups who benefit from treatment even if others, perhaps the majority, do not. The problem lies in identifying these subgroups of children when they present; while we can observe the heterogeneity, we have so far been unable to explain it convincingly.

There is a well established principle amongst advocates of RCTs that if a significant and clinically important effect is observed for a study population as a whole, the direction of the effect is extremely unlikely to reverse for any subgroup although the size of the effect may vary (Peto et al., 1993). This principle is used to argue that trials within subgroups are rarely needed, and that subgroup analyses within trial populations should not be performed. This principle cannot be applied so confidently in reverse, i.e. if no effect is observed in a study population as a whole, it remains possible that there could be a clinically important effect for a subgroup of the population.

Following a recent systematic review of preschool vision screening (Snowdon and Stewart-Brown, 1997), which concluded that there was no high quality evidence of the effectiveness of occlusion treatment, there is increasing pressure for RCTs of occlusion. In this context, it is important to consider how a finding of no clinically important effect of treatment from a trial powered to detect a difference in a heterogeneous population would be interpreted. There seems to me to be a real danger of concluding that occlusion is not effective for all, when there may be a clinically important benefit in one or more subgroups. Ideally, any RCT should be large enough to have adequate power for subgroup analyses, with randomization stratified by relevant subgroups. The 'Catch 22' is that relevant subgroups have not yet been identified.

One should not overlook other, practical problems that are likely to arise with a RCT. In view of the established nature of occlusion therapy, I suggest that it is important to establish that equipoise exists amongst parents and practitioners before committing substantial resources to a RCT; otherwise there are likely to be problems recruiting and the results will have poor applicability. Care needs to be taken to avoid contamination and other biases. The inability to mask patients and parents to the treatment might introduce bias when measuring outcome, even if the orthoptist or researcher responsible for recording outcome is masked. Ideally, a persuasive alternative (but ineffective) treatment is required for the control group to exclude a placebo effect. Few trials are perfect in every respect and I do not intend to imply that these problems are insurmountable; they are, however, formidable, and are likely to contribute to the difficulty of interpreting the results of a RCT.

CONCLUSIONS

Amblyopic patients appear to constitute a heterogenous population. Relevant subgroups with respect to prognosis/outcome of treatment have not been clearly identified. In these circumstances, there are dangers in carrying out a pragmatic RCT evaluation.

What then should the immediate clinical research agenda be? In view of our relative ignorance of natural history, I suggest that what we need immediately are high quality, prospective, large cohort studies. Because of the naturally occurring variation in occlusion practices, such studies may also contribute some information about interactions between treatment and subgroups. These studies should, as far as possible, adopt research quality standards with respect to data collection. Such studies are often criticized for being a data 'trawl' when there are no clear *a priori* hypotheses. This is a legitimate criticism, but I maintain that the approach is justifiable in view of our current ignorance. Findings from such studies should be viewed cautiously in the short term, and be re-tested as *a priori* hypotheses of interest in new or continuing cohorts. This approach does not preclude concurrent RCTs, since these could be nested amongst cohort studies in contributing centres where equipoise exists (Black, 1999).

A second item on the research agenda should be the stability of visual acuity improvements achieved by treatment. Valid studies of this topic could almost certainly be carried out retrospectively by centres with good records of previously treated patients. A related but separate theme should be the disability experienced by amblyopes in adult life; this theme is addressed in detail in Chapter 6.

A final item on the research agenda relates to the properties of measurements, e.g. test–retest reliability and inter-observer agreement, for many of the operational criteria that are used to define amblyopia. Retrospective reviews of case notes suggest that these signs have a habit of coming and going, although it is not clear whether this intra-subject variation arises as a result of measurement error by the observer or true fluctuation over time. Studies of these measurement properties are simple to do, and yet are sadly absent from the literature. In one sense these are the most urgent studies of all, since, until we can quantify the uncertainty of the measurements that underpin our descriptions of amblyopia, it will be hard to make definitive progress on the other research agenda items.

REFERENCES

Abrahamsson, M. and Sjöstrand, J. (1996). Natural history of infantile anisometropia. *Br. J. Ophthalmol.*, **80**, 860–63.

Abrahamsson, M., Fabian, G. and Sjöstrand, J. (1992). Refraction changes in children developing convergent or divergent strabismus. *Br. J. Ophthalmol.*, **76**, 723–7.

Almeder, L. M., Peck, L. B. and Howland, H. C. (1990). Prevalence of anisometropia in volunteer laboratory and school screening populations. *Inv. Ophthalmol. Vis. Sci.*, **31**, 2448–55.

Attebo, K., Mitchell, P., Cumming, R. *et al.* (1998). Prevalence and causes of amblyopia in an adult population. *Ophthalmology*, **105**, 154–9.

Begg, C., Cho, M., Eastwood, S. *et al.* (1996). Improving the quality of reporting of randomized controlled trials: the CONSORT statement. *J. Am. Med. Assoc.*, **276**, 637–9.

Black, N. (1996). Why we need observational studies to evaluate the effectiveness of health care. *Br. Med. J.*, **312**, 1215–18.

Black, N. (1999). High-quality clinical databases: breaking down barriers. *Lancet*, **353**, 1205–6.

Catford, J. C., Absolon, M. J. and Millo, A. (1984). Squints – a sideways look. In: *Progress in Child Health*, Vol. 1 (J. A. Macfarlane, ed.), pp. 38–49. Churchill Livingstone.

Chalmers, I. and Altman, D. G. (eds) (1995). *Systematic Reviews*. BMJ Publishing Group.

Chalmers, I., Hetherington, J., Elbourne, D. *et al.* (1989). Materials and methods used in synthesizing evidence to evaluate the effects of care during pregnancy and childbirth. In: *Effective Care in Pregnancy and Childbirth* (I. Chalmers, ed.), pp. 39–65. Oxford University Press.

Ciuffreda, K. J., Levi, D. M. and Selenow, A. (1991). *Amblyopia: Basic and Clinical Aspects*. Butterworth-Heinemann.

Elwood, M. (1998). *Critical Appraisal of Epidemiological Studies and Clinical Trials*, 2nd edn. Oxford University Press.

Fielder, A. R. and Moseley, M. J. (1996). Anisometropia and amblyopia – chicken or egg? *Br. J. Ophthalmol.*, **80**, 857–8.

Flynn, J. T. and Cassady, J. C. (1978). Current trends in amblyopia therapy. *Ophthalmology*, **85**, 428–50.

Hardman Lea, S. J., Loades, J. and Rubinstein, M. P. (1989). The sensitive period for anisometropic amblyopia. *Eye*, **3**, 783–90.

Helveston, E. M. and von Noorden, G. K. (1967). Microtropia: a newly defined entity. *Arch. Ophthalmol.*, **78**, 272–81.

Hiscox, F., Strong, N., Thompson, J. R. *et al.* (1992). Occlusion for amblyopia: a comprehensive survey of outcome. *Eye*, **6**, 300–304.

Ingram, R. M., Holland, W. W., Walker, C. *et al.* (1986). Screening for visual defects in pre-school children. *Br. J. Ophthalmol.*, **70**, 16–21.

Jaeschke, R. and Sackett, D. L. (1989). Research methods for obtaining primary evidence. *Int. J. Tech. Assess. Healthcare*, **5**, 503–19.

Kheterpal, S., Jones, H. S., Auld, R. and Moseley, M. J. (1996). Reliability of visual acuity in children with reduced vision. *Ophthal. Physiol. Optics*, **16**, 447–9.

Kohler, L. and Stigmar, G. (1973). Vision screening of four-year-old children. *Acta Paediatr. Scand.*, **62**, 17–27.

Lithander, J. and Sjöstrand, J. (1991). Anisometropic and strabismic amblyopia in the age group 2 years and above: a prospective study of the results of treatment. *Br. J. Ophthalmol.*, **75**, 111–16.

NHS Management Executive (1992). *Assessing the Effects of Health Technologies*. Department of Health.

Peto, R., Collins, R. and Gray, R. (1993). Large-scale randomized evidence: large, simple trials and overviews of trials. *Annals NY Acad. Sci.*, **703,** 314–40.

Schapero, M. (1971). *Amblyopia.* Chilton.

Snowdon, S. K. and Stewart-Brown, S. L. (1997). *Preschool Vision Screening: Results of a Systematic Review.* NHS Centre for Reviews and Dissemination.

Stayte, M., Johnson, A. and Wortham, C. (1990). Ocular and visual defects in a geographically defined population of 2-year-old children. *Br. J. Ophthalmol.*, **74,** 465–8.

Stayte, M., Reeves, B. and Wortham, C. (1993). Ocular and vision defects in preschool children. *Br. J. Ophthalmol.*, **77,** 228–32.

Thompson, J. R., Woodruff, G., Hiscox, F. A. *et al.* (1991). The incidence and prevalence of amblyopia detected in childhood. *Public Health*, **105,** 455–62.

von Noorden, G.K. (1985). *Binocular Vision and Ocular Motility. Theory and Management of Strabismus*, 3rd edn. C. V. Mosby Co.

Woodruff, G., Hiscox, F., Thompson, J. R. and Smith, L. K. (1994a). The presentation of children with amblyopia. *Eye*, **8,** 623–6.

Woodruff, G., Hiscox, F., Thompson, J. R. and Smith, L K. (1994b). Factors affecting the outcome of children treated for amblyopia. *Eye*, **8,** 627–31.

5 Amblyopia: treatment and evaluation

Merrick Moseley

INTRODUCTION

An historical consideration of amblyopia treatment would undoubtedly conclude this topic to be long on innovation yet short on critical evaluation (see Table 5.1). Consider the following remark by Paliaga (1997):

> To an unbiased observer the amblyopia treatment domain could appear to be a sort of privileged enclosure exempt from the obligation to apply the methodological rules universally adopted in clinical research concerning treatment of other diseases.

The message here is that amblyopia treatment appears – to adopt modern parlance – to be insufficiently evidence-based. But to what extent is this true? Figure 5.1 provides a list of primary and secondary study designs rank-ordered according to the 'hierarchy of evidence' (see Greenhalgh, 1997). The position of a particular study design within this hierarchy defines the relative

Table 5.1 Amblyopia treatments by category. For historical reviews see Unwin (1991) and Ciuffreda *et al.* (1991). Italicized treatments are reviewed in this chapter

Physical	Electrotherapy
	Light/pattern stimulation
	Massage
	Occlusion
	Penalization
	Refractive correction
Pharmacological	Barbiturates
	Neuromodulators/neurotransmitter precursors
	Strychnine
	Vasodilators
Psychological	Hypnosis
Dietary	Veal and red wine

Figure 5.1 *'Hierarchy of evidence' (after Greenhalgh, 1997).*

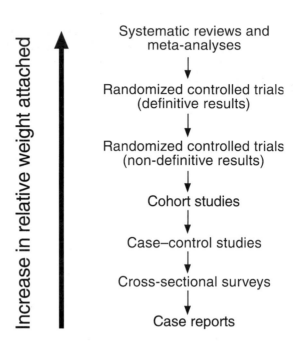

weight given to research findings when treatment decisions come to be made. If all the published literature on amblyopia treatment were to be classified on this basis, then pictorially this would resemble a somewhat bottom-heavy pyramid with perhaps just one systematic review at its apex.

Whilst it is accepted that all new treatments should be subject to rigorous evaluation (preferably to the level of a randomized controlled trial, RCT), there is a rational debate as to the need to evaluate treatments established within clinical practice prior to the advent of the evidence-based approach. On the one hand there is a concern not to 'reinvent the wheel' – it is unlikely that one would gain funding or ethical approval to evaluate immobilization for the treatment of simple bone fracture. Yet on the other hand we know the history of therapeutic medicine to be replete with examples where the effectiveness of numerous treatments remained undisputed until shown otherwise by determined sceptics. Where do amblyopia treatments fit into this scheme? Certainly, many would regard a prospective RCT of occlusion therapy as a pointless exercise. Such opinion though sits uneasily with the findings of the only systematic review of this topic, which firmly concludes that just such a study should be undertaken (Snowdon and Stewart-Brown, 1997a). This review asserted that whilst there was sufficient evidence '. . . to substantiate beliefs that children with amblyopia do improve during treatment . . .', it judged that '. . . this evidence falls very far short of showing that treatment works'. Lack of knowledge of the natural history of amblyopia was identified as the causal link between these seemingly contradictory statements, although a combination of Hawthorne, practice and placebo effects are all capable of exerting their influence where deficiencies in study designs permit.

Justified though it may be, the expressed need for controlled treatment trials should not rule out other important strands of scientific enquiry. This is perhaps stating the obvious but, as will be seen, there are many questions, not least amongst the most established treatments, that are worthy of investigation.

This chapter has been written with the aim of drawing to the attention of the reader developments in amblyopia treatment occurring in the last 10 years or so. It is not a guide to management, and nor is it a systematic review of the research literature. Rather, it seeks to identify where research efforts are currently focused and the problems within these areas that present specific challenges.

CURRENT STATUS AND RECENT DEVELOPMENTS

Pharmacological treatments

Levodopa

Awareness of the role of dopamine as a neurotransmitter and its observed depletion in the retinae of visually deprived animals led Gottlob and Stangler-Zuschrott (1990) to undertake the first reported study of amblyopia treatment with this neurotransmitter precursor. In a single-dose (220 mg, oral) placebo-controlled trial, they demonstrated in nine adult amblyopes statistically significant improvements in visual acuity and contrast sensitivity, and a reduction in fixation point scotomas. The functional improvements arising from single-dose administration of levodopa were later confirmed by Leguire and colleagues (1992) in amblyopic children unresponsive to occlusion therapy. The previously noted side effects of levodopa administration, typically nausea and emesis, could be reduced with appropriate attention to dosage, although this did impact on the reported acuity gains (Leguire et al., 1993a).

Several trials of levodopa have subsequently been published (Gottlob et al., 1992; Leguire et al., 1993a, 1993b) in all of which statistically (if not functionally) significant outcomes have been reported, often in comparison to placebo controls and in combination with occlusion therapy. None, however, seem to have recruited children presenting with previously untreated amblyopia.

Levi (1994) reanalysed the data of Leguire et al. (1995), comparing the rate of change (slope) of improvement seen in the amblyopic and placebo groups and finding them not to differ significantly from one another. On the basis of this observation, and further that levodopa did not appear to produce improvements (whether functional or significant) beyond that expected by occlusion, Levi concluded that: ' . . . it seems unlikely that levodopa will alter the 200-year-old tradition of occlusion therapy'. Whilst occasional reports of levodopa use continue to appear (Gottlob et al., 1995; Leguire et al., 1995, 1998; Basmak et al., 1999; Procianoy et al., 1999), Levi's remarks seem to have been borne out by the passage of time. There has been little progress in identifying those patients who might benefit most from levodopa, or indeed to treat those children who present for the first time in early childhood, or to establish the long-term stability of any treatment gains. Levodopa clearly does not *cure* amblyopia, and it is unclear if, even in combination with occlusion therapy, the additional benefits really merit this neuropharmacological intervention with its added risks and costs.

Citicoline

Citicoline (cytidine–5′-diphosphocholine) is an endogenous molecule, the obligate intermediary for the synthesis of phosphatidylcholine, and a major phospholipid in the plasma membrane. Its predominant therapeutic use to date has been to raise consciousness levels in neurological disease. It is also thought to increase the availability of certain neuromodulators and neuro-transmitters, including dopamine – hence its use as a complement to levodopa therapy in Parkinson's disease. Other tentative clinical roles include the treatment of glaucoma (Giraldi *et al.*, 1989; Parisi *et al.*, 1999). Laboratory studies of visual function in adult amblyopes indicates that citicoline can improve visual acuity and contrast sensitivity and augment the visual evoked potential (Porciatti *et al.*, 1998).

Campos and co-workers were the first (and currently the only) group to have described the treatment of amblyopia using citicoline (Campos *et al.*, 1995). They argued that residual plasticity speculated to exist in the adult amblyopic visual system might be activated by the administration of this drug. They report both an uncontrolled (UCT) and a randomized placebo-controlled trial (RCT) of citicoline on a total of 60 patients with anisometropic, strabismic and deprivational amblyopia (UCT, $n = 50$; RCT, $n = 10$; age, 9–37 years). The drug regimen consisted of daily doses of 1000 mg i.m. citicoline (physiological solution in RCT placebo controls) for 15 days. Linear and single letter acuities were recorded weekly during the first month, then monthly for up to 18 months. Linear acuity improved by a mean of approximately 0.18 log units (UCT) and 0.22 log units (RCT). There were no improvements seen in the placebo group of the RCT.

In a further study, Campos and colleagues (Campos *et al.*, 1997) reported the effects of citicoline in a group of older child amblyopes aged from 5–9 years (thought able to tolerate i.m. administration at a reduced dose of 500 mg daily for 10 days repeated at 6 months) who had previously undergone occlusion therapy. Subjects were randomized to three treatment groups: citicoline (A); citicoline plus minimal occlusion (1 hour/day) (B); and minimal occlusion only (C). Average treatment gains at 1 year for linear acuity were 0.325 log units in group A, 0.276 log units in group B, and 0.160 log units in group C. Treatment gains in groups A and B were shown to be significantly greater ($P < 0.001$) than those seen in group C. The authors emphasized the additional benefits of combining citicoline with occlusion therapy (group B) in that 4 months after the start of treatment (2 months prior to the second administration of citicoline) the rate of improvement in this group was maintained, whereas in the citicoline-only group (A) improvement had ceased – albeit temporarily.

This latter study establishes that treatment of children with citicoline leads, without reported side effects, to gains in acuity comparable to those seen in adults. Unfortunately, the lack of a placebo control leaves open to doubt the therapeutic mechanism that may have been operating in this study. Campos *et al*. acknowledge the practical difficulties of i.m. drug administration in children, and point out that although the oral route of administration is permissible, dosage regimens have yet to be standardized.

That citicoline acts by stimulation of the dopaminergic system accords with the observation that in all studies where citicoline has been administered to amblyopic subjects, gains in acuity were also manifest in the fellow eye (i.e. non-specific action). However, citicoline's neuropharmacological actions are not confined to dopaminergic stimulation, and, given that the clinical status of the fellow eye in amblyopia is ambiguous (see following section), one cannot rule out alternative modes of action of this drug.

Correction of refractive error

It is unusual for a definition of a disease to include its unresponsiveness to a particular treatment. However, many definitions of amblyopia make note of the fact that the visual deficit cannot be ameliorated by optical correction. Paradoxically, the importance of establishing a focused retinal image has always been stressed in amblyopia management. Traditionally, 'active' treatment is carried out in parallel with, or proceeds from, the correction of any refractive error. In this paradigm, refractive correction serves only to optimize a defective visual system from an optical standpoint and plays no role in reversing the residual visual loss – i.e. the amblyopia. However, it is not implausible to suggest that the provision of high spatial frequency information arising from refractive correction to a visual system previously deprived of such will facilitate neural activity, leading to an increase in visual resolution (for a possible explanation of mechanisms underpinning such activity, see Mitchell and Gingras, 1998). Such a notion has been tacitly accepted for some time, gains in acuity occurring over a period of weeks after refractive correction but before 'active' treatment being sometimes loosely attributed to 'spectacle adaptation'. Some go further, asserting that refractive correction may be actively therapeutic in the treatment of anisometropic amblyopia (see e.g. Kivlin and Flynn, 1981), but such gains remain poorly quantified.

It can of course be argued that it is the final outcome of treatment that is of importance, and not the individual contribution of the various components. There are, however, valid reasons why it is important to analyse the benefits of refractive correction separately from those of, say, occlusion. First, we are reasonably certain that spectacle wear is far more tolerable than occlusion, and therefore if use of the former negates the need for the latter, then this must be considered clinically worthy. Secondly, where after spectacle wear residual amblyopia remains, necessitating occlusion, it can be argued that a lesser amount might be required and that this will be better tolerated than had it been instigated before any gains due to spectacle wear had been realized. Thirdly, in any treatment trial it is essential that performance gains attributable to refractive correction be distinguished from those arising from the treatment under evaluation.

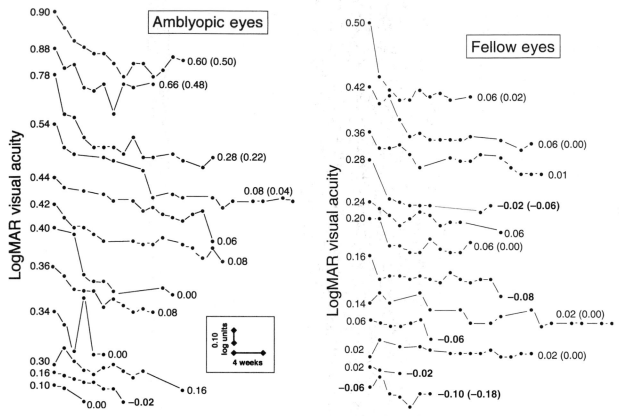

Figure 5.2 *'Waterfall' plot of logMAR visual acuity as a function of time (amblyopic eyes). Each line represents the relative change in visual acuity of a single subject. Initial and final corrected acuities appear, respectively, on the left and right of each plot. Parenthetic values are best acuities attained during study if not those recorded at last visit.*

Figure 5.2 illustrates an attempt to quantify the improvements that might be expected to occur in the visual acuity of amblyopic children prescribed only spectacle wear. None of the 12 children, aged from 3.8 to 6.3 years, had received previous treatment, all having been diagnosed with 'straight-eyed' amblyopia with two having the additional association of esotropia. Linear logMAR visual acuity was recorded whenever possible at weekly intervals in both amblyopic and fellow eyes until acuity had stabilized according to an algorithm based upon the number of inflexions in the plot of acuity versus time.

The striking feature of the plots is that the improvement appears universal; no subject failed to make gains in acuity, which ranged from 0.1 to 0.5 log units over a period of 4 to 25 weeks. Eight of the subjects did not require any subsequent treatment, having attained within 0.1 log units of 'normal' (0.0 logMAR) acuity.

Interestingly, improvements ranging from 0.02 to 0.32 log units were also seen in subjects' fellow eyes. This observation has some implication for the likely mechanism(s) underpinning the acuity gains seen – perhaps initially suggesting that a simple practice effect might lie at the heart of the improvements. To examine this possibility, we recruited and tested six subjects (aged 4.1–6.8 years) in a manner identical to that already described, excepting that acuity was recorded initially with the newly prescribed refractive correction and then again seven weeks later without any intervening measurements. The changes in acuity seen in these subjects (range 0.08–0.60 log units) are at least comparable to those seen at 7 weeks in the initial study. These findings suggest that practice effects cannot account for the time-dependent improvements seen when an amblyopic eye is optically corrected, and that some alternative mechanism must be implicated.

A close inspection of the data shown in Figure 5.2 reveals that although gains in acuity continued to a maximum of 22 weeks, no subject improved by more than 0.1 log units beyond 18 weeks. Such a period is one that might routinely be adopted as a suitable period of 'spectacle adaptation' (spectacle treatment?) before additional amblyopia therapy is contemplated. That improvements in the fellow eye are seen which cannot easily be deemed to have arisen from practice raises the issue of whether the fellow eye is indeed a normal eye. Such a conjecture is in keeping with the presence of subtle, fellow-eye defects demonstrated on psychophysical tasks (e.g. see Wali *et al.*, 1991; Woo and Irving, 1991).

Penalization

As a descriptive term, penalization has been deemed 'singularly odd' but nonetheless '. . . an effective alternative to occlusion treatment . . .' (von Noorden, 1990). Introduced into clinical practice by the French School in the nineteenth century, it appears to have entered routine practice early the next (see Worth, 1903). In the latter twentieth century its use seems to have dwindled to the point at which Repka and Ray (1993) felt it necessary to state, as a goal of their study, the need to '. . . acquaint ophthalmologists with its ease of administration and efficacy . . .'. More recently, though, penalization has been subject to evaluation in prospective and retrospective trials, which may herald its renaissance into practice if initially promising results are confirmed.

Penalization can be effected by optical, pharmacological or combined means, with the objective of degrading near vision (or more rarely distance vision, or both) in the fellow eye. Several advantages of penalization over occlusion are claimed. Stereopsis may still operate during treatment whilst a full binocular visual field is maintained, although whether this is of any real significance remains, in the opinion of LaRoche (1998), 'unproven'. A further claimed advantage of penalization over occlusion is that it cannot evoke latent nystagmus.

Implicit in the therapeutic principle underpinning penalization is that the fellow eye be sufficiently penalized to ensure fixation is maintained at near in the amblyopic eye. LaRoche (1998) notes a general tendency for this matter to be ignored in reports of the effectiveness of penalization. Recently, however, Wallace (1999) has empirically derived data which, taking into account the visual acuity of the amblyopic eye and the refractive error of the fellow eye, can be used as means to determine *a priori* whether penalization should be considered an appropriate treatment.

A trend apparent in the most recent publications is for pharmacological (i.e. atropine) penalization to be favoured over that of optical penalization. This is perhaps unsurprising given its simplicity and certainty of near absolute compliance. An interesting development here is that of a so-called 'inter-mittent' regimen of penalization, where the traditional daily application is reduced to one to three drops (depending upon iris colour) of atropine per week. The claimed advantages of this reduced administration are that it offers some protection against the occurrence of reverse amblyopia (allowing greater intervals between assessments), presents less need to maintain an exact correction in the better eye, and is more manageable for the care giver. Retrospective analyses have shown the intermittent regimen to be of equivalent effectiveness to traditional, full-time atropine penalization (Simons *et al.*, 1997a, 1997b).

It is argued that a child's world is a near world, and in order for penalization to be effective (at least by its claimed mechanism) this observation must necessarily be true. Yet there appears to be little quantitative data on this in the amblyopia literature (certainly the 'developmental psychology' literature has not been raided by the advocates of penalization to support their claims). We are left therefore to go along with the (not unreasonable) statement by Worth (1903) that 'A young child spends at least half his waking hours in looking at near objects', which he goes on to equate with '. . . perfect occlusion of the "fixing eye" for at least half of each day'. This does however seem to be an over-simplistic view (forgivable perhaps for one held at the beginning of the twentieth century, but not at the start of the twenty-first) where it should be possible, given a reliable estimate of a child's looking behaviour, to model the effect of penalization as spatio-temporal filtering. One thing we can be sure of, however, is that penalization is not simply part-time occlusion by other means.

The effectiveness of penalization (i.e. the achievement of statistically significant post treatment improvements in visual acuity) has been demonstrated up to the level of a controlled trial (Doran *et al.*, 1990), where its effectiveness was established as being equivalent to that of occlusion. Therapeutic equivalence with occlusion therapy has been confirmed in retrospective and prospective cohort studies (Foley-Nolan *et al.*, 1997; Simons *et al.*, 1997a, 1997b). A large ($n = 400$) randomized trial of penalization versus occlusion funded by the US National Eye Institute (Amblyopia Treatment Study, ATS1) is currently underway, which should provide the strongest indication to date of the relative effectiveness of these two treatments.

Occlusion therapy

In general, we tend not to reflect on the fact that occlusion therapy is a generic term used to describe what is in reality a series of disparate treatment regimens. It can be applied to either eye, be partially or totally occluding (to form vision), and be prescribed according to a multiplicity of doses (from 'minimum' to 'full-time'). Whilst recent years have not seen any new variants on traditional (full-time, part-time) treatment regimens emerge, some attention has been given to patch construction with a view to compliance monitoring (see, 'Measurement of compliance and dose').

Presently, the prime topic of interest is treatment evaluation first mooted in the late 1980s (Fulton and Mayer, 1988) and given impetus with the emerging focus on evidence-based medicine in the 1990s. This has finally emerged as a research priority (at least in the UK) by the publication of the NHS CRD report of a systematic review of pre-school vision screening (Snowdon and Stewart-Brown, 1997a). Several research groups have taken up this challenge, adopting a variety of approaches to treatment evaluation, including those of pragmatic randomized controlled trials (RCTs) and dose–response studies.

There follows a brief review of planned or in-progress studies known to the author. It is not claimed to be exhaustive, but should provide the reader with an indication of current activity in this area and the potential utility of the findings that may arise.

Monitored Occlusion Treatment for Amblyopia Study (MOTAS)

The principal investigators in this study are M. J. Moseley and A. R. Fielder, of the Imperial College School of Medicine, London, UK.

This study differs from those subsequently discussed in that it does not adopt any of the epidemiological study designs that make up the 'traditional hierarchy of evidence' (Figure 5.1). MOTAS sets out to define dose–response functions for occlusion where, in broad terms, dose is defined as the amount of occlusion (duration and temporal occurrence) and response is the change in visual function (logMAR visual acuity, stereo acuity, letter contrast sensitivity). This statistical modelling approach is used extensively in the analysis of drug trials and toxicology (see Chuang-Stein and Agresti, 1997). The rationale for the adoption of this unusual (for 'fully-fledged' treatments) study design is that so little is known of the kinetics of occlusion (stemming in large part from the hitherto impossibility of accurate compliance measurement) that it would be inadvisable to proceed to non-pragmatic RCTs of occlusion when we have no knowledge of what regimens might be worthy of inclusion. Put at its simplest, if dose–response studies indicate that occlusion for periods of, say, 4 hours a day yields performance gains that do not differ from those of, say, 8 hours per day, then it would be inappropriate to include within a future RCT 8 hours occlusion/day as a candidate regimen. MOTAS should be viewed as a precursor of conventional treatment evaluation whose designs will no doubt be greater informed by its outcome.

Implicit in the approach adopted by MOTAS is the requirement for accurate and objective measurement of treatment compliance (occlusion dose). All subjects enrolled in the study will be patched in conjunction with an occlusion dose monitor (see 'Measurement of compliance and dose'). One notable aspect of this study is that prior to the prescription of occlusion (which all

Table 5.2 Summary of study design: Monitored Occlusion Treatment of Amblyopia Study (MOTAS)

Study design	Three-phase, multi-site study of dose–response (see text); Phase 1: assessment, consent, enrolment; Phase 2: spectacle wear (if indicated); Phase 3: occlusion
Subjects	120
Treatment	Phase 1: 18 weeks spectacle wear (if indicated); Phase 2: continuation of spectacle wear (where prescribed in phase 1) + 6 hours occlusion per day until acuity stable or participants no longer meet acuity entry criterion
Duration	24 months initially
Principal inclusion criteria	Aged 3.5–7 years at recruitment; newly identified with amblyopia associated with anisometropia, strabismus or both; acuity deficit in amblyopic eye ≥ 0.1 logMAR and interocular difference ≥ 0.1 log units
Principal exclusion criteria	Learning difficulties or mental retardation; ocular pathology including amblyopia associated with form deprivation
Principal outcome measures	Distance logMAR acuity (Keeler acuity cards, modified ETDRS charts); letter contrast sensitivity (Pelli–Robson chart); objective measurement of occlusion using Occlusion Dose Monitor (see text)
Comments	Variations in occlusion dose arise from expectation of variable compliance

subjects are initially scheduled to undergo), children who on study entry present with clinically significant refractive errors will undergo an 18-week period of spectacle wear to ensure that gains in performance attributable to spectacle adaptation are not falsely attributed to the subsequent occlusion (see 'Correction of refractive error').

The experimental design of MOTAS is summarized in Table 5.2.

Randomized Controlled Trial of Treatment of Unilateral Straight-Eyed Visual Acuity Deficit

The principal investigators in this study are M. Clarke and C. Wright, of the University of Newcastle-upon-Tyne, UK.

This study is a pragmatic, multi-centre RCT with three treatment arms: occlusion, spectacle wear, and a no-treatment control group. The inclusion of the latter is an innovation not reported in any recent amblyopia treatment trial, and adds considerably to the power of the experimental design. However, the inclusion of a no-treatment arm has, as one might expect given the mainstream status of occlusion, not been without its critics (Simons and Preslan, 1999; see Appendix). In defence, it should be pointed out that the trial excludes all children with latent or manifest squints and includes only those straight-eyed amblyopes with mild acuity deficits.

Outcome measures are limited solely to uncorrected logMAR visual acuity tested at 6 and 12 months after enrolment and corrected acuity at 12.5 months. The adoption of *uncorrected* acuity as a principal outcome is a significant feature of the design which allows the straightforward optical benefits of refractive correction to be distinguished from those of either longer-term spectacle wear or of longer-term spectacle wear combined with occlusion.

Other noteworthy features of this experimental design include the use of treatment diaries to be kept by parents of children entered into the occlusion arm of the study. Additionally, all parents of enrolled children will be invited to complete a 'family impact questionnaire', which, irrespective of the main outcome, will additionally provide an indication as to whether occlusion has negative consequences for family life – a factor which, though asserted, has been to a major extent unstudied (Snowdon and Stewart-Brown, 1997b; Stewart-Brown and Snowdon, 1998).

A summary of the experimental design of this RCT is provided in Table 5.3.

Table 5.3 Summary of study design: Randomized Controlled Trial of Treatment of Unilateral Straight-Eyed Visual Acuity Deficit

Study design	Pragmatic, multi-site randomized controlled trial with no treatment arm; masked assessment at 6 and 12 months (uncorrected); unmasked assessment (corrected) at 12.5 months
Subjects	220
Treatment	Group 1: no treatment; Group 2: spectacle wear if indicated; Group 3: spectacle wear if indicated + occlusion therapy (initially 180 minutes per day of fellow eye, then 90–360 minutes per day depending on acuity gains seen at interim assessments)
Duration	30 months
Principal inclusion criteria	Aged 3–4 years at recruitment; newly identified with 'straight-eyed' amblyopia; acuity deficit in amblyopic eye in range 6/9–6/36
Principal exclusion criteria	Manifest and latent strabismus; significant developmental delay
Principal outcome measures	LogMAR acuity (Keeler acuity cards), family impact questionnaire
Comments	Compliance with occlusion and spectacle wear monitored using parental diaries

Amblyopia Treatment Study 'ATS2' (US)

The ATS Protocol Chairman is J. Holmes, The Mayo Clinic, MN, USA, and this study is being conducted under the auspices of the Pediatric Eye Disease Investigator Group (PEDIG).

This multi-centre RCT will compare the effectiveness of part-time versus full-time occlusion in a sample of amblyopic children with the key inclusion criterion of severe amblyopia (amblyopic eye acuity in the range 0.8–1.3 logMAR). The focus on severe amblyopia arises from the observation that occlusion therapy is presently considered the only appropriate initial treatment for these cases. The comparison of full-time (all, or all but 1 of waking hours) versus part-time (6 hours per day) is proposed, as there is conflicting anecdotal evidence as to their relative effectiveness. Proponents of full-time patching would claim that restoration of visual acuity can be achieved more rapidly this way, whilst those advocating part-time occlusion claim that this regimen produces less stress on the parent–child relationship, better compliance, and the promotion of binocularity in 'straight-eyed' amblyopes.

There is clearly a strong pragmatic component in this trial, as, due to non-compliance, the occlusion doses actually received by the children may end up being only marginally different between the two treatment groups. Indeed, many European practitioners might define 6 hours daily occlusion

Table 5.4 Summary of study design: Amblyopia Treatment Study (ATS2)

Study design	Randomized, controlled, single-masked, multi-centre
Subjects	160
Treatment	Refractive correction for a minimum of 4 weeks (if indicated); part-time occlusion (6 hours per day); full-time occlusion (all day or all but 1 waking hour per day)
Duration	24 months
Principal inclusion criteria	Aged <7 years (but not in or within 4 months of entering 1st grade); visual acuity testable using single, surrounded HOTV on BVAT; amblyopia associated with anisometropia, strabismus or both; amblyopic eye acuity in range <20/125–≥20/400; fellow eye acuity ≥20/40
Principal exclusion criteria	No or limited amblyopia treatment in the preceding 6 months; ocular disease (excluding nystagmus); previous intraocular surgery
Principal outcome measures	LogMAR acuity (single-surrounded HOTV (BVAT)) at 4 months and 24 months; Amblyopia Treatment Index (a 20-item quality of life questionnaire administered to the primary care giver)
Comments	Compliance with occlusion monitored using caregivers' diaries (log)

as full- rather than part-time therapy. However, if no difference emerges between the relative effectiveness of the two treatment groups whilst at the same time the supplied caregivers' diaries show little evidence that the received occlusion dose differed greatly between groups, then this would provide strong evidence that, at least *in practice*, full-time occlusion offers no advantage over a part-time regimen.

A summary of the experimental design of the Amblyopia Treatment Study is provided in Table 5.4.

TREATMENT EVALUATION

Outcome variables

Vision scientists now recognize that the amblyopic visual system, once solely characterized by a loss of visual acuity, manifests a cluster of deficits across many visual subsystems, including *inter alia* the pupillary, the accommodative and the oculo-motor systems (Ciuffreda *et al.*, 1991; McKee *et al.*, 1992). In contrast, routine clinical practice generally relies solely on visual recognition acuity either of optotypes present in isolation ('single letter') or linear arrays ('linear acuity') as the principal treatment metric. However, in the course of formal evaluation of amblyopia treatments, is it valid to rely on such simple traditional measures? In considering this question, it is important to be aware of the varying objectives of different strands of amblyopia research. Here, an important distinction needs to be made between a *laboratory* study, in which the aim is to quantify the visual deficit independent of any concurrent treatment regimen (see, for example, Chapter 2), and a *clinical study*, in which changes in visual function are recorded sequentially over the course of a particular treatment regimen. In the laboratory, there is much greater freedom to determine the subjects' visual function on a gamut of visual tests structured over one or more sessions. This situation contrasts strikingly with an attempt to evaluate changes in visual performance as a function of treatment where visual testing must be incorporated into the overall treatment plan. In this situation, subjects (who for the most part will be young children) must not be overburdened less their performance deteriorate due to fatigue. Thus, in the context of evaluation of amblyopia therapy, there is definitely mileage in the adage 'it is better to test a few functions well, than many badly'.

In this chapter we are concerned with treatment evaluation (in a clinical context), and in this field there have been no suggestions that any attributes of visual performance be assessed other than those of spatial visual function. Thus discussion here will be reserved to the following: visual acuity (single, crowded and positional) and contrast sensitivity.

Visual acuity

Distance visual acuity recorded with shapes or letter optotypes remains the *de facto* standard means of defining the spatial deficit in amblyopia and as an outcome measure by which treatment is monitored routinely or as part of a treatment evaluation. It is a relatively simple test to administer and has high face validity as an index of seeing ability. In the past few decades considerable attention has been given to the use of appropriately scaled tests of visual acuity (see Westheimer, 1979), which has led to increased use of optotypes scaled according to the logarithm of the minimum of angle of resolution (logMAR). The practical, theoretical and statistical advantages of logMAR charts over the traditional Snellen (reciprocal MAR) charts can be found elsewhere (Moseley and Jones, 1993; McGraw et al., 1995). LogMAR charts are available in single letter, linear, and linear crowded formats, and have been used successfully to monitor the visual deficit of amblyopic patients undergoing treatment (Moseley et al., 1997; Simmers et al., 1999).

Positional acuity, usually recorded in the form of a vernier alignment task ('vernier acuity') has a long tradition as a laboratory test of amblyopic vision. In general, vernier acuity is regarded as the most sensitive measure of the amblyopic deficit (i.e. one in which the greatest magnitude of deficit will be recorded relative to the norms of other measures of spatial visual performance), although this is not universally true (see Simmers and Gray, 1999). A vernier or other positional acuity task for use among child amblyopes has in theory excellent potential, and could perhaps be incorporated into an electronic game format for automated testing.

Visual acuity testing has also assumed a quasi-diagnostic significance with the development of the repeat letter test chart (Regan et al., 1992), which seeks to discriminate between amblyopia associated with abnormal gaze control and that associated with abnormal eye movements. With the exception of a single adult study, repeat letter testing does not seem to have yet found favour as an outcome measure per se in treatment evaluation studies.

Contrast sensitivity

Whilst it is recognized that visual acuity in general offers a useful index of seeing ability, it nonetheless provides only a sparse description of the visual system's ability to process spatial information. The contrast sensitivity function (CSF) (Campbell and Green, 1965) provides a more comprehensive measure having a characteristic band-pass appearance in normal observers whilst being, to varying degrees, low pass in amblyopic observers (see Ciuffreda et al., 1991 and Chapter 2).

To determine an observer's CSF, a series of threshold measurements are obtained across a range of spatial frequencies for a given target (generally cosine gratings). This fact immediately places constraints on the measurement of contrast sensitivity in treatment trials, where, as already remarked upon, test duration is a significant issue. To some extent this problem is not solely one associated with the testing of children in a clinical context, but indeed with contrast sensitivity testing in all routine clinical situations. To this end it has been argued that it may be sufficient to test a restricted number of spatial frequencies (Pelli et al., 1988; Wilkins et al., 1988). The argument goes along the lines that given, at its simplest level, the choice of testing at either low, medium or high spatial frequencies, it is judged inappropriate to test at high spatial frequencies (on the grounds that such a measure may be highly correlated with visual acuity) and likewise at low spatial frequencies (on the grounds that deficits in this region are a rarity), thus leaving only the medium spatial frequency region as a plausible indicator of visual sensitivity that may reveal a spatial deficit not otherwise identified by traditional visual acuity measures.

Drawing upon this argument, several tests of contrast sensitivity have been developed that seek to provide a measure of contrast sensitivity in the medium (2–4 c/deg region) either using gratings (Wilkins *et al.*, 1988) or letter optotypes (Pelli *et al.*, 1988).

Defining an appropriate test battery

Our choice of outcome measure(s) should not be primarily directed at characterizing the nature of the visual disturbance, but rather on its usefulness in monitoring change. Following on from this assumption leads us to reflect on the extent to which outcome measures might be correlated in practice. If measures of two separate visual functions are correlated across time (treatment duration), it must be suspected that both reflect the same underlying factors and thus (at least for the purposes of treatment evaluation) one must be considered redundant.

This phenomenon is clearly indicated in the findings of Simmers and co-workers (1999). These authors recorded the changes occurring in a single amblyopic patient as a function of treatment duration on six spatial visual tasks (Figure 5.3). Whilst it can be seen that performance on each task differs

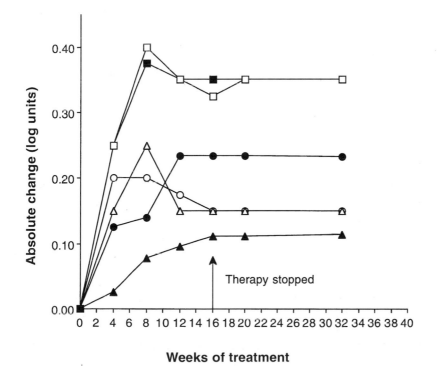

Figure 5.3 *Comparison of improvements in visual function of an adult amblyope during occlusion therapy. Upward arrow indicates cessation of therapy. Open squares, repeat letter acuity; filled squares, crowded letter acuity; open circles, single letter acuity; filled circles, oscillatory motion displacement thresholds; open triangles, low contrast letter acuity; closed triangles, alignment thresholds. From Simmers and Gray (1999), reproduced with permission.*

for both pre- and post-treatment measures, there exists a considerable degree of correlation in the improvement seen as treatment progresses. This study was a single case history of an adult patient, where it was in the researchers' interest to explore the usefulness of all the available tests. However, given the observed level of correlation it would be difficult to justify the inclusion of such a variety of visual tasks within a treatment trial with the knowledge that they may not be tapping unique characteristics of amblyopic visual function.

Mindful of an over-reliance upon visual acuity testing, Moseley and co-workers (1997) included letter contrast sensitivity within their test battery for use in a pilot study of amblyopia treatment effectiveness. They adopted the Pelli–Robson chart, on the basis that it provides a measure of sensitivity to the mid-range of spatial frequencies and that it complemented the adopted test of visual acuity by employing the same letter set. However, these authors observed an almost one-to-one non-parametric correlation between logMAR acuity and letter contrast sensitivity, which hints at the redundancy of contrast sensitivity measurement at least for the target and spatial frequency test region provided by the Pelli–Robson chart. In the MOTAS study (see 'Occlusion therapy') the authors have chosen initially to include letter contrast sensitivity in the test battery, although should evidence of its redundancy again be found its use will be discontinued.

Functional outcomes

In choosing appropriate treatment outcome measures, it is natural to consider, in the first instance, the clinical and psychophysical tests with which we have a ready familiarity. However, we need to be reminded that: 'The ideal outcome of treatment is a return to the normal or usual quality of life for a given age or medical condition' (Jenkinson and McGee, 1997). Thus we can conceive of a hierarchy of outcomes. At the bottom we have simple – in the case of amblyopia – psychophysical indicators of outcome. At one step up the hierarchy we can record visual performance at real world visual tasks e.g. navigation, manipulation of tools; and at the top of the hierarchy, self-assessment of quality of life.

To date, outcome measures of amblyopia treatment have exclusively relied upon relatively simple psychophysical measures. Given our present state of knowledge this reliance is perhaps an excusable one, although it should be possible to record outcomes according to an appropriately standardized, age-normed, complex visual-motor task once we have a better understanding of how the various component skills for such tasks (e.g. acuity, stereopsis) are themselves influenced by treatment.

As for the impact of amblyopia treatment on quality of life, it is heartening to see that measurement of this is being undertaken in certain of those controlled trials (ATS2, Randomized Controlled Trial of Treatment of Unilateral Straight-Eyed Visual Acuity Deficit) as previously described. As for the effect of amblyopia *per se* on quality of life in adulthood, one unfortunately runs into problems of a quasi-philosophical nature – those questioned being unable to draw upon any experience of life without amblyopia. Notwithstanding these difficulties, there have been recent attempts (Snowdon and Stewart-Brown, 1997b; Packwood *et al.*, 1999; see also Chapter 6) to do just this.

Compliance and dose

Although the meaning of the terms *compliance* and *dose* would seem straightforward in a general medical context, their use is not without controversy. In the case of the former, arguments have been put forward that it might better be replaced by the arguably less authoritarian term *concordance* (Mullen, 1997). Here I have chosen not to adopt this term, as for the most part I shall be making reference to literature that predates its use.

Although the term *dose* is used in a standard sense when pharmacological treatments for amblyopia are referred to, it is seldom used as a descriptor of an occlusion regimen. This is unfortunate, because I believe there is much to be gained by emphasizing the analogy between drug regimens (in general) and occlusion regimens. It is indeed biologically plausible, not to say taken for granted by most practitioners, that the amount of occlusion is in some way related to treatment outcome – in other words, there will exist a *dose–response relationship*. Further, it can be hypothesized that the period over which a given amount of occlusion occurs (*dose rate*) will also have some bearing on outcome. As previously argued, I believe there are valid grounds for examining the dose–response relationship of occlusion therapy, which is both a prerequisite analysis and complementary approach to accepted methods of treatment evaluation such as the RCT.

Among the principal factors thought to influence the outcome of occlusion therapy (e.g. age, severity, category of amblyopia), any systematic review would undoubtedly flag-up treatment compliance as being of crucial significance (see e.g. Oliver *et al.*, 1986; Lithander and Sjöstrand, 1991; Nucci *et al.*, 1992; Mintz-Hittner and Fernandez, 2000). Indeed, historically, seemingly barbaric practices such as eyelid suture (Weckert, 1932) and arm splinting (Hiles and Galket, 1974) have been prescribed in order to ensure absolute compliance.

Although occlusion therapy is a highly aversive experience (as just a few minutes experience of self-patching will confirm!), it would be wrong to attribute inadequate compliance solely to this single factor. Undoubtedly non-compliance has multifactorial origins, including poor awareness of the rationale and urgency of the treatment, cosmetic appearance, and parental stress. Sadly the investigation of compliance with patch wear has been sorely neglected, although there are encouraging signs that it may now be receiving the attention it deserves with the publication of two recent reports (Newsham, 2000; Searle *et al.*, 2000) tackling the problem from a health psychology perspective.

Measurement of compliance and dose
Although compliance is widely held to be a major factor influencing treatment outcome, it should be borne in mind that until relatively recently only subjective

(e.g. treatment diary, parental interview) and crude, objective measures of treatment compliance (e.g. clinic attendance) were available. Intriguingly, one of the few studies to have undertaken detailed objective compliance monitoring (Fielder *et al.*, 1995) actually observed, albeit in a single subject, significant gains in visual performance where compliance was meagre!

There is undoubtedly a need for precise, objective measurements of occlusion, and the devices required in order to undertake this are now important research tools that may one day find a place in routine clinical practice. Before considering these in more detail, let us briefly consider the pros and cons of alternative measures of compliance.

Almost all routine estimates of compliance are gleaned from parental interview. Clearly, one can only expect to gain crude qualitative data by this means, and in addition there is the obvious bias that interviews of this nature tend to elicit information which the interviewee perceives will satisfy the (clinician) interviewer (Cramer, 1991). A refinement of the parental interview is the use of an occlusion diary, again a subjective method and also prone to bias. Notwithstanding problems of legibility and the sometimes lengthy time required to translate diary entries into a readily manipulatable format such as a spreadsheet, quantitative information can be elicited (Fielder *et al.*, 1995; see also Moseley and Fielder, 1996). Parental diaries are currently employed in some of the treatment trials already described. Whilst numerically crude, clinic attendance does at least have the virtue of objectivity and has been used to differentiate, retrospectively, compliant and non-compliant subjects (Nucci *et al.*, 1992).

Promisingly, more sophisticated means of objective measurement are now available. The first 'occlusion dose monitor' (ODM) was introduced by Fielder and co-workers in 1994. A modified version of the original device (Figure 5.4) is being used in the MOTAS study (Table 5.2) in an attempt to determine the dose–response characteristics of occlusion therapy in amblyopic children. Briefly, the ODM consists of a data logging unit and a modified, disposable occlusion patch. The battery-operated logging unit connects via a lead (usually concealed under the child's clothes) to the patch, whose undersurface contains electro-conductive materials. The logging unit records all episodes of patch–skin contact (sampling resolution typically 60s). On return to the clinic, the ODM is connected to a PC and the occlusion time-history downloaded for analysis. In practice, parents have little difficulty in administering the ODM; it has no patient/parent-operated controls and requires only that a simple plug-in connection be made between the logging unit and the patch.

Simonsz and co-workers (1999) have also described an occlusion dose monitor in which episodes of patch wear are logged electronically. In their design, patch–skin contact is inferred by the existence of a temperature differential across the internal and external surfaces of the occlusive patch (Figure 5.5), with the logging unit and patch integrated into a single unit. The lack of any connecting lead is an apparent ergonomic advantage (*cf.* Figure 5.4), but this has to be offset against the risk that the logging unit may be inadvertently disposed of when the patch is removed.

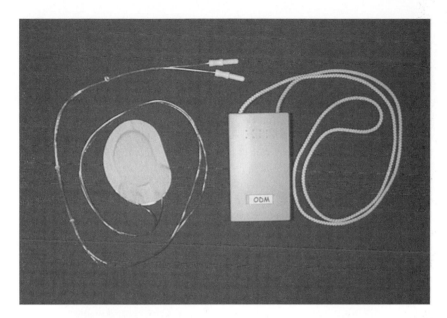

Figure 5.4 *Occlusion dose monitor (Fielder et al., 1994): Device detects electrical resistance across miniature electrodes positioned on patch undersurface (see text).*

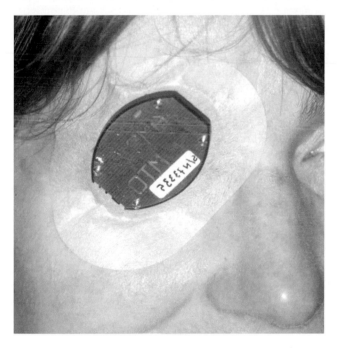

Figure 5.5 *Occlusion dose monitor (Simonsz et al., 1999). Device detects temperature differential sensed between internal and external surfaces (see text). Reproduced with permission of authors.*

THE TREATMENT OF OLDER CHILDREN AND ADULTS

Several factors set the agenda for this topic. First, and most obviously, adult patients present far less frequently than children. Secondly, predominant clinical opinion is such that treatment in this age group is unlikely to be successful, such judgements being based to a varying degree on personal experience perhaps underpinned by notions of critical or sensitive periods derived from animal models. However, the literature on this topic is equivocal (Garzia, 1987; Ciuffreda *et al.*, 1991; Wick *et al.*, 1992; Levi, 1994; Mintz-Hittner and Fernandez, 2000). Levi (1994) makes a plea against a simplistic approach, arguing that the age of onset of amblyopia is a more critical parameter than that of age of onset of treatment, and draws upon Worth's classic study (Worth, 1903) to illustrate this point. Levi concludes that failure to achieve improvement does not imply a lack of plasticity and that '. . . it may, rather, reflect the very real difficulties in maintaining patient (or clinician) motivation . . .', but acknowledges that this viewpoint contradicts current clinical dogma. Latterly, Levi and co-workers (Levi *et al.*, 1997) have shown that adult amblyopes demonstrate perceptual learning of positional acuity, implying the presence of residual plasticity in the adult amblyopic visual system. Indeed, in this study involving thousands of trials of a positional acuity task, there was clear evidence that this effect had transferred to recognition (Snellen) acuity where dramatic improvements were seen, albeit in a small number of subjects. Most recently, Polat and Ma-Naim (2001) have described a perceptual learning-based treatment paradigm based on the detection of Gabor targets. Among a group of 47 adult amblyopes (9–55 years), mean gains in distance letter acuity of 0.2 ± 0.25 log units were attained over twenty 30-minute sessions. Only negligible gains (0.02 log units) were apparent in a control group.

One recent case report on this topic is particularly worthy of note insofar as the authors report (Simmers and Gray, 1999) the outcome of a battery of visual function tests (including single letter, crowded, low contrast and hyperacuity). Their subject was a 30-year-old strabismic amblyope who had had his application for a Heavy Goods Vehicle (HGV, truck) licence declined. The subject was described as highly motivated and underwent 16 weeks of part-time occlusion (3–4 hrs/day). At the end of treatment, improvement was apparent in all of the visual functions recorded ranging from 23–55% (just over three lines in the case of logMAR acuity), and gains appeared to be maintained up to 32 weeks. The subject was ultimately able to obtain his licence and pursue his new occupation. The authors conclude that future research is required to investigate the efficacy of amblyopia treatment in adults. Given a not insubstantial evidence base, albeit mostly at the level of case reports, and the recent evidence of plasticity in the amblyopic visual system, this claim, it is hoped, will be heeded. Indeed ATS3 (*cf.* ATS1, ATS2) will be examining the effectiveness of occlusion in 7–18-year-olds (J. Holmes, personal communication).

CONCLUSIONS

Sadly, the history of amblyopia treatment research is for the most part one of passing fads and unsubstantiated claims. The enormous gains in the understanding of the physiological and psychophysical basis of the condition (see elsewhere in this monograph) appear not to have made a commensurate impact on the treatment offered to patients. Researchers and clinicians venturing into this area need to be mindful of the Confucian adage: 'a wise man knows how little he knows'.

Occlusion therapy at the turn of the millennium retains its status as the mainstream treatment of choice, yet only after many decades during which the opportunity existed are concerted attempts now being made to evaluate its effectiveness. New pharmacological treatments will necessarily undergo stringent evaluation before their place in the clinic becomes established, as will treatments said to be undergoing a revival, such as penalization. Notwithstanding the arguments that occlusion should have been more rigorously evaluated earlier, at least we now have some useful tools to assist us: improved tests of visual function and the means to monitor objectively the amount of occlusion patients receive.

Whilst all acknowledge that amblyopia is a developmental disorder and that early treatment remains a primary concern, the consequences of amblyopia may be experienced in adulthood. At a basic level, inadequately treated amblyopia may lead to a restriction in career opportunities due to a failure to meet statutory occupational vision standards (see Adams and Karas, 1999 for a discussion), and the risk of visual disability arising from loss of function in the fellow eye (see e.g. Tommila and Tarkkanen, 1981; Rahi *et al.*, 2000; Chapter 6) remains a concern. Yet although there exist numerous reports of treatment success in adults, clinical dogma and scepticism has until very recently downgraded this as a research priority. Meanwhile, there exists a strand of opinion that deems the use of occlusion therapy in childhood is sufficiently traumatic to patient and family that its worthiness is suspect.

This chapter has been written at a time when a far more questioning attitude to amblyopia treatment is becoming mainstream. Whilst many of us may in time be disappointed that practices we once advocated will turn out to be of limited value, only by continuing our research efforts to generate, refine and evaluate treatments can we expect benefits to patients to be forthcoming.

ACKNOWLEDGEMENTS

I would like to thank Jonathan Holmes for his constructive criticism of this chapter and for information relevant to the PEDIG studies described herein, and Mike Clarke, who openly provided details of the Newcastle study. Thanks also to Kurt Simons for his enjoyably combative transatlantic emails.

REFERENCES

Adams, G. G. W. and Karas, M. P. (1999). Effect of amblyopia on employment prospects. *Br. J. Ophthalmol.*, **83**, 380.

Basmak, H., Yildirim, N., Erdinc, O. *et al.* (1999). Effect of levodopa therapy on visual evoked potentials and visual acuity in amblyopia. *Ophthalmologica*, **213**, 110–13.

Campbell, F. W. and Green, D. G. (1965). Optical and retinal factors affecting visual resolution. *J. Physiol.*, **181**, 576–93.

Campos, E. C., Schiavi, C., Benedetti, P. *et al.* (1995). Effect of citicoline on visual acuity in amblyopia: preliminary results. *Graefe's Arch. Clin. Exper. Ophthalmol.*, **233**, 307–12.

Campos, E. C., Bolzani, R., Schiavi, C. *et al.* (1997). Cytidin–5′-diphosphocholine enhances the effect of part-time occlusion in amblyopia. *Documenta Ophthalmologica*, **93**, 247–63.

Chuang-Stein, C. and Agresti, A. (1997). Tutorial in biostatistics. A review of tests for detecting a monotone dose-response relationship with ordinal response data. *Stat. Medicine*, **16**, 2599–618.

Ciuffreda, K. J., Levi, D. M. and Selenow, A. (1991). *Amblyopia: Basic and Clinical Aspects*. Butterworth-Heinemann.

Cramer, J. A. (1991). Overview of methods to measure compliance and enhance patient compliance. In: *Patient Compliance in Medical Practice and Clinical Trials*. (J. A. Cramer and B. Spilker, eds), pp. 3–10. Raven Press.

Doran, R. M. L., Yarde, S. and Starbuck, A. (1990). Comparison of treatment methods in strabismic amblyopia. In: *Strabismus and Ocular Motor Disorders*. (E. C. Campos, ed.), pp. 51–9. Macmillan Press.

Fielder, A. R., Auld, R., Irwin, M. *et al.* (1994). Compliance monitoring in amblyopia therapy. *Lancet*, **343**, 547.

Fielder, A. R., Irwin, M., Auld, R. *et al.* (1995). Compliance monitoring in amblyopia therapy: objective monitoring of occlusion. *Br. J. Ophthalmol.*, **79**, 585–9.

Foley-Nolan, A., McCann, A. and O'Keefe, M. (1997). Atropine penalisation versus occlusion as the primary treatment for amblyopia. *Br. J. Ophthalmol.*, **81**, 54–7.

Fulton, A. B. and Mayer, D. L. (1988). Esotropic children with amblyopia: effects of patching on acuity. *Graefe's Arch. Clin. Exper. Ophthalmol.*, **226**, 309–12.

Garzia, R. P. (1987). Efficacy of vision therapy in amblyopia: a literature review. *Am. J. Optom. Physiol. Optics*, **64**, 393–404.

Giraldi, J. P., Virno, M., Covelli, G. *et al.* (1989). Therapeutic value of citicoline in the treatment of glaucoma (computerized and automated perimetric investigation). *Int. Ophthalmol.*, **13**, 109–12.

Gottlob, I. and Stangler-Zuschrott, E. (1990). Effect of levodopa on contrast sensitivity and scotomas in human amblyopia. *Inv. Ophthalmol. Vis. Sci.*, **31**, 776–80.

Gottlob, I., Charlier, J. and Reinecke, R. D. (1992). Visual acuities and scotomas after one week levodopa administration in human amblyopia. *Inv. Ophthalmol. Vis. Sci.*, **33**, 2722–8.

Gottlob, I., Wizov, S. S. and Reinecke, R. D. (1995). Visual acuities and scotomas after 3 weeks' levodopa administration in adult amblyopia. *Graefe's Arch. Clin. Exper. Ophthalmol.*, **233**, 407–13.

Greenhalgh, T. (1997). *How to Read a Paper*. BMJ Publishing Group.

Hiles, D. A. and Galket, R. J. (1974). Plaster cast arm restraints and amblyopia therapy. *J. Ped. Ophthalmol.*, **11**, 151–2.

Jenkinson, C. and McGee, H. (1997). Patient assessed outcomes: measuring health status and quality of life. In: *Assessment and Evaluation of Health and Medical Care* (C. Jenkinson, ed.), pp. 64–84. Open University Press.

Kivlin, J. D. and Flynn, J. T. (1981). Therapy of anisometropic amblyopia. *J. Ped. Ophthalmol. Strab.*, **18**, 47–56.

LaRoche, G. R. (1998). Detection, prevention, and rehabilitation of amblyopia. *Curr. Opin. Ophthalmol.*, **9**, 10–14.

Leguire, L. E., Rogers, G. L., Bremer, D. L. *et al.* (1992). Levodopa and childhood amblyopia. *J. Ped. Ophthalmol. Strab.*, **29**, 290–98.

Leguire, L. E., Rogers, G. L., Bremer, D. L. *et al.* (1993a). Levodopa/carbidopa for childhood amblyopia. *Inv. Ophthalmol. Vis. Sci.*, **34**, 3090–95.

Leguire, L. E., Walson, P. D., Rogers, G. L. *et al.* (1993b). Longitudinal study of levodopa/carbidopa for childhood amblyopia. *J. Ped. Ophthalmol. Strab.*, **30**, 354–60.

Leguire, L. E., Walson, P. D., Rogers, G. L. *et al.* (1995). Levodopa/carbidopa treatment for amblyopia in older children. *J. Ped. Ophthalmol. Strab.*, **32**, 143–51.

Leguire, L. E., Rogers, G. L., Walson, P. D. *et al*. (1998). Occlusion and levodopa–carbidopa treatment for childhood amblyopia. *J. Am. Assoc. Ped. Ophthalmol. Strab*., **2**, 257–64.

Levi, D. M. (1994). Pathophysiology of binocular vision and amblyopia. *Curr. Opin. Ophthalmol*., **5**, 3–10.

Levi, D. M., Polat, U. and Hu, Y.-S. (1997). Improvement in vernier acuity in adults with amblyopia. Practice makes better. *Inv. Ophthalmol. Vis. Sci*., **38**, 1493–1510.

Lithander, J. and Sjöstrand, J. (1991). Anisometropic and strabismic amblyopia in the age group 2 years and above: a prospective study of the results of treatment. *Br. J. Ophthalmol*., **75**, 111–16.

McGraw, P., Winn, B. and Whitaker, D. (1995). Reliability of the Snellen chart. *Br. Med. J*., **310**, 1481–2.

McKee, S. P., Schor, C. M., Steinman, S. B. *et al*. (1992). The classification of amblyopia on the basis of visual and oculomotor performance. *Trans. Am. Ophthalmol. Soc*., **90**, 123–48.

Mintz-Hittner, H. A. and Fernandez, K. M. (2000). Successful amblyopia therapy initiated after age 7 years: compliance cures. *Arch. Ophthalmol*., **118**, 1535–41.

Mitchell, D. E. and Gingras, G. (1998). Visual recovery after monocular deprivation is driven by absolute, rather than relative, visually evoked activity levels. *Curr. Biol*., **8**, 1179–82.

Moseley, M. J. and Fielder, A. R. (1996). Occlusion therapy for childhood amblyopia: current concepts in treatment evaluation. In: *Infant Vision* (F. Vital-Durand, J. Atkinson and O. J. Braddick, eds), pp. 383–99. Oxford University Press.

Moseley, M. J. and Jones, H. S. (1993). Visual acuity: calculating appropriate averages. *Acta Ophthalmol. (Copenh.)*, **71**, 296–300.

Moseley, M. J., Fielder, A. R., Irwin, M. *et al*. (1997). Effectiveness of occlusion therapy in ametropic amblyopia: a pilot study. *Br. J. Ophthalmol*., **81**, 956–61.

Mullen, P. D. (1997). Compliance becomes concordance. *Br. Med. J*., **314**, 691–2.

Newsham, D. (2000). Parental non-concordance with occlusion therapy. *Br. J. Ophthalmol*., **84**, 957–62.

Nucci, P., Alfarano, R., Piantanida, A. and Brancato, R. (1992). Compliance in antiamblyopia occlusion therapy. *Acta Ophthalmol. (Copenh.)*, **70**, 128–31.

Oliver, M., Neumann, R., Chaimovitch, Y. *et al*. (1986). Compliance and results of treatment for amblyopia in children more than 8 years old. *Am. J. Ophthalmol*., **102**, 340–45.

Packwood, E. A., Cruz, O. A., Rychwalski, P. J. and Keech, R. V. (1999). The psychosocial effects of amblyopia study. *J. Am. Assoc. Ped. Ophthalmol. Strab*., **3**, 15–17.

Paliaga, G. P. (1997). Major review: controversies in functional amblyopia. *Binoc. Vision Strab. Q*., **12**, 155–66.

Parisi, V., Manni, G., Colacino, G. and Bucci, M. G. (1999). Cytidine–5′-diphosphocholine (citicoline) improves retinal and cortical responses in patients with glaucoma. *Ophthalmology*, **106**, 1126–34.

Pelli, D. G., Robson, J. G. and Wilkins, A. J. (1988). The design of a new letter chart for measuring contrast sensitivity. *Clin. Vision Sci*., **2**, 187–99.

Polat, U. and Ma-Naim, T. (2001). Treatment of adult amblyopia by perceptual learning. *Inv. Ophthalmol. Vis. Sci*., **42**, S400.

Porciatti, V., Schiavi, C., Benedetti, P. *et al*. (1998). Cytidine–5′-diphosphocholine improves visual acuity, contrast sensitivity and visually-evoked potentials of amblyopic subjects. *Curr. Eye Res*., **17**, 141–8.

Procianoy, E., Fuchs, F. D., Procianoy, L. and Procianoy, F. (1999). The effect of increasing doses of levodopa on children with strabismic amblyopia. *J. Am. Assoc. Ped. Ophthalmol. Strab*., **3**, 337–40.

Rahi, J. S., Logan, S., Timms, C. *et al*. (2000). Incidence and causes of new visual loss affecting the non-amblyopic eye of individuals with unilateral amblyopia in the United Kingdom. *Inv. Ophthalmol. Vis. Sci*., **41**, S296.

Regan, D., Giaschi, D. E., Kraft, S. P. and Kothe, A. C. (1992). Method for identifying amblyopes whose reduced line acuity is caused by defective selection and/or control of gaze. *Ophthal. Physiol. Optics*, **12**, 425–32.

Repka, M. X. and Ray, J. M. (1993). The efficacy of optical and pharmacological penalization. *Ophthalmology*, **100**, 769–75.

Searle, A., Vedhara, K., Norman, P. *et al*. (2000). Compliance with eye patching in children and its psychosocial effects: a qualitative application of protection motivation theory. *Psychol. Health Med.*, **5**, 43–54.

Simmers, A. J. and Gray, L. S. (1999). Improvement of visual function in an adult amblyope. *Optom. Vision Sci.*, **76**, 82–7.

Simmers, A. J., Gray, L. S., McGraw, P. V. and Winn, B. (1999). Functional visual loss in amblyopia and the effect of occlusion therapy. *Inv. Ophthalmol. Vis. Sci.*, **40**, 2859–71.

Simons, K. and Preslan, M. (1999). Natural history of amblyopia owing to lack of compliance. *Br. J. Ophthalmol.*, **83**, 582–7.

Simons, K., Gotzler, K. C. and Vitale, S. (1997a). Penalization versus part-time occlusion and binocular outcome in treatment of strabismic amblyopia. *Ophthalmology*, **104**, 2156–60.

Simons, K., Stein, L., Sener, E. C. *et al*. (1997b). Full-time atropine, intermittent atropine, and optical penalization and binocular outcome in treatment of strabismic amblyopia. *Ophthalmology*, **104**, 2143–55.

Simonsz, H. J., Polling, J. R., Voorn, R. *et al*. (1999). Electronic monitoring of treatment compliance in patching for amblyopia. *Strabismus*, **7**, 113–23.

Snowdon, S. K. and Stewart-Brown, S. L. (1997a). *Preschool Vision Screening: Results of a Systematic Review*. NHS Centre for Reviews and Dissemination.

Snowdon, S. K. and Stewart-Brown, S. L. (1997b). *Amblyopia and Disability: A Qualitative Study*. Health Services Research Unit, University of Oxford.

Stewart-Brown, S. and Snowdon, S. K. (1998). Evidence-based dilemmas in pre-school vision screening. *Arch. Dis. Child.*, **78**, 406–7.

Tommila, V. and Tarkkanen, A. (1981). Incidence of loss of vision in the healthy eye in amblyopia. *Br. J. Ophthalmol.*, **65**, 575–7.

Unwin, B. (1991). The treatment of amblyopia – a historical review. *Br. Orthop. J.*, **48**, 28–31.

von Noorden, G. K. (1990). *Binocular Vision and Ocular Motility*, 4th edn. C. V. Mosby Co.

Wali, N., Leguire, L. E., Rogers, G. L. and Bremer, D. L. (1991). CSF interocular interactions in childhood amblyopia. *Optom. Vision Sci.*, **68**, 81–7.

Wallace, D. K. (1999). Visual acuity after cycloplegia in children: implications for atropine penalization. *J. Am. Assoc. Ped. Ophthalmol. Strab.*, **3**, 241–4.

Weckert, H. (1932). Neue Wege zur Bekämpfung der Schielamblyopie. *Zentralbl. Ophthalmol. Grenzgebiete*, **27**, 239.

Westheimer, G. (1979). Scaling of visual acuity measurements. *Arch. Ophthalmol.*, **97**, 327–30.

Wick, B., Wingard, M., Cotter, S. and Scheiman, M. (1992). Anisometropic amblyopia: is the patient ever too old to treat? *Optom. Vision Sci.*, **69**, 866–78.

Wilkins, A. J., Della Sala, S., Somazzi, L. and Nimmo-Smith, I. (1988). Age-related norms for the Cambridge low contrast gratings, including details concerning their design and use. *Clin. Vision Sci.*, **2**, 201–12.

Woo, G. C. and Irving, E. (1991). The non-amblyopic eye of a unilateral amblyope: a unique entitity. *Clin. Exper. Optom.*, **74**, 1–5.

Worth, C. (1903). *Squint: Its Causes, Pathology, and Treatment*. John Bale, Sons & Danielsson, Ltd.

6 Amblyopia and disability

Alistair Fielder

INTRODUCTION

Intuitively, one would assume that having two eyes functioning normally and in synchrony is crucial to human well-being; after all the brain has installed a highly complex wiring system just so that this happens. So highly prized is the resultant binocular vision that massive amounts of health service resources worldwide are poured into the early identification and treatment of any deficits of binocular function in children.

Pursuing this theme, it is also intuitive that impairment of one eye, so that binocular vision is disrupted, would impart a disability. One such condition is childhood amblyopia. However, the assumption that the impairment associated with amblyopia causes disability has recently been questioned. Consider the following statements taken from two influential reports:

> Unfortunately, we have little or no explicit data concerning the impact of amblyopia on quality of life measures, such as limitations in an individual's ability to complete activities of daily living, the impact of amblyopia on career opportunities or choices.
>
> (Hartmann, 1999)

> There is lack of good quality research into the natural history of the target conditions {amblyopia, refractive errors and squint}, the disabilities associated with them, and the efficacy of available treatments . . . In the absence of sound evidence that the target conditions sought in these programmes are disabling and that the interventions available to correct do more good than harm, the ethical basis for such interventions is very insecure.
>
> (Snowdon and Stewart Brown (1997)

So while binocular vision is thought to exemplify the highest level of visual functioning, its loss appears to carry with it no significant or even identifiable disability, and its treatment (by occlusion) may have a negative impact exceeding that of the amblyopia itself.

In this chapter, I will address the impact of amblyopia on quality of life. In the absence of explicit data, I will first discuss the benefits of having two eyes, before specifically considering disability. Inevitably, the frequent association of amblyopia with strabismus and refractive error necessitates that these conditions also be factored into the equation.

THE BENEFITS OF HAVING TWO EYES

Stereopsis and other visual functions

There are a number of benefits of having two as opposed to one normally functioning eye (see Fielder and Moseley, 1996; Westlake, 2001). Binocular concordance (probability summation from the receipt of largely matched monocular information) underpins the superiority of binocular over monocular acuity (Blake and Fox, 1973; Jones and Lee, 1981) rather than stereopsis (receipt of mismatched monocular information).

Stereopsis, that is the binocular perception of depth based upon retinal disparity (Bishop, 1987) is generally accepted to be the major advantage of having two eyes. By reducing the amount of scanning required to extract spatial information stereopsis facilitates comprehension of complex visual experiences, so providing efficient access to information on depth in our surroundings (Wickens *et al.*, 1994). Monocular cues can also provide information indirectly on depth through linear perspective, shadows, texture and gradients etc. However, stereopsis provides the only *direct* source of depth information (Bishop, 1987; Westheimer, 1992), and it is possible that secondary cues, themselves dependent on retinal disparity, are able to substitute in part for stereopsis.

Stereopsis results from the integration of two slightly dissimilar retinal images. It is affected by contrast, illumination, colour, texture and stimulus presentation time (Bishop, 1987; Stuart *et al.*, 1992; Westheimer, 1992; Johnston *et al.*, 1993; Wickens *et al.*, 1994). The distance over which stereopsis operates is probably up to about 100 metres, and it improves as the distance reduces until it becomes limited by accommodation (Bishop, 1987; von Noorden, 1990; Cartmill, 1992; Snyder and Lezotte, 1993).

Stereopsis emerges between about 3 and 5 months of age (Birch, 1993), and adult levels of 30–40 seconds of arc (Westheimer, 1992) are reached by the age of 5–7 years (Simons, 1981, 1993; Heron *et al.*, 1985). Infrequently, stereoblindness occurs in asymptomatic adults with no other disorder of binocular function; otherwise abnormal stereopsis occurs in ophthalmic conditions that disrupt binocular vision in childhood, and also in a range of neurological disorders.

Many authors have sung the praises of stereopsis – consider: '. . . highest form of binocular cooperation which adds a new quality to vision . . .' (von Noorden, 1990); '. . . provides a vivid and accurate relative depth experience' (Bishop, 1987); 'Stereo acuity is considered as a bench mark for peak clinical performance of binocular vision' (Schor, 1991). However, this view is not held by all: 'Nature gave us two eyes so that one is spare . . . Stereoscopic vision is of little value except in a few occupations' (Phillips, 1987). This latter position was robustly attacked by Sir George Godber, who had lost one eye many years previously, noting '. . . a long held personal suspicion that few ophthalmologists know the full consequences of total loss of vision in one eye' (Godber, 1987). Even three decades after the loss of an eye, Godber reported, as have others (Brady, 1985), misjudging distances, problems with hand–eye coordination, and perceptual difficulties so that 'To the one-eyed golfer all greens are flat' (Godber, 1987).

Whilst a number of professions have exacting visual requirements, the functional implications of not achieving these levels for the tasks required by these occupations is largely unknown. It has been suggested that stereopsis does not correlate with flying ability, and that under most conditions monocular cues suffice. However, in unfamiliar and stressful conditions stereopsis might be beneficial, for example in assessing ground proximity and adverse weather conditions (Snyder and Lezotte, 1993)! Similarly, comparing stereo-normal and stereo-abnormal motorists, stereopsis was found to improve driving performance only in dynamic situations at intermediate distances (Bauer et al., 2000). Utilizing a simple test of manual dexterity – threading a loop along a bent wire, as encountered at village fêtes – the skills of stereo-normal ophthalmic surgeons were compared to other professionals with and without stereopsis (Murdoch et al., 1991). Ophthalmologists performed the task significantly better than non-ophthalmologists both with and without stereopsis, and the non-ophthalmologists with good stereopsis were significantly better than those with no stereopsis, but not better than those with reduced stereopsis. Burden, an ophthalmic surgeon with strabismus (but presumably not amblyopia) has described how he '. . . learned alternative methods of achieving depth perception . . .' so that, in his opinion, his surgical expertise was unimpaired (Burden, 1994).

Clinical evidence

Bax and Whitmore (1973), in a study of 657 school entrants, observed that children with strabismus had significantly higher neurodevelopmental scores (i.e. more abnormal) than the 'average'. Alberman and co-workers (1971) also observed, in the National Child Development Study of 15 496 children, that the prevalence of cerebral palsy, neurodevelopmental delay or clumsiness with strabismus was higher than in controls. Children with strabismus but without neurodevelopmental problems still performed less well as readers and at copying design than controls. Wheeler et al. (1979) did not observe a change on developmental scales after strabismus surgery, although an improvement of binocular-dependent motor skills occurred in 35 per cent of children after correction of infantile esotropia (Rogers et al., 1982).

Strabismus has a negative psychosocial effect in childhood that may increase in teenage and adult life (Satterfield et al., 1993). Parents of children who had undergone surgical correction of strabismus under the age of 4 years reported a number of benefits such as: improved eye contact, better interaction with others and raised self-esteem. Coordination was deemed by parents to be improved in 56 per cent of cases (Mruthyunjaya *et al.*, 1996).

Recently the psychosocial effects of amblyopia in individuals without strabismus has been studied (Packwood *et al.*, 1999). The 25 study patients (aged 15–64 years) reported interference with the following: education (52 per cent); work (48 per cent); lifestyle to some degree (50 per cent); and sport (40 per cent). In addition, individuals with amblyopia experienced more distress in areas of somatization, obsession–compulsion, interpersonal sensitivity, anxiety and depression compared to controls. Packwood *et al.* (1999) compared their results with those obtained from individuals with strabismus (data of Satterfield *et al.*, 1993) and failed to detect a significant difference. Stewart-Brown *et al.* (1985) noted reduced intelligence among those with amblyopia and reduced reading skills associated with mild hypermetropia; spectacle wear did not affect scores. Patients with defective vision of only one eye (not reduced by amblyopia have lower associated quality of life compared to those with good vision in both eyes (Brown *et al.*, 2001).

Expansion of the visual field by 8–30 degrees following surgery for a convergent strabismus was noted (Kushner, 1994) regardless of the presence of amblyopia. As drivers with field loss are reported to have an increased risk of being involved in an accident, this finding is important (Keltner, 1994). Powerful clinical evidence for the importance of good binocular function comes from the functional benefit adults gained from second eye cataract surgery in a randomised controlled trial (Laidlaw *et al.*, 1998). In this study there were major benefits to patients, attributed to improved stereoacuity, which could not otherwise be explained on the basis of gains in visual acuity or contrast sensitivity.

Strabismus is well known to be associated, as has frequently been reported, with neurodevelopmental problems. However, the picture emerging does not clarify in any way whether strabismus causes motor incoordination, or whether both are the consequence of a subtle neurological insult. In addition, no study has been designed to tease out the relationship, with respect to disability, between amblyopia, strabismus and refractive status.

Experimental evidence

When reviewing experimental (non-clinical) approaches to investigating the functional significance of binocular vision, one needs to be mindful that stereopsis is operational in the near, rather than the far, distance. The first approach focuses on depth judgement as exemplified by the work of Wickens *et al.* (1994), who showed that 3-D representation facilitated and accelerated visualization of a complex surface, possibly by making viewing judgements more precise, and by reducing both effortful scanning and searching. Interestingly, the process itself was not more accurate, and there was no long-term retention of this knowledge.

The second experimental approach is to investigate the motor response required by a skilled task, especially in one that requires complex hand–eye coordination. Sensory input has a critical role in fine motor control (Lemon,

1999), and involves the transfer of visual information from parietal to premotor areas (Jeannerod *et al.*, 1995) to create links between vision, cognition and action. Milner and Goodale (1996) have proposed that there are separate processes for visual perception (ventral stream) and transforming visual information into motor action (dorsal stream). While the structure and function of these streams is not fully delineated, both arise from the visual cortex, and they have parvocellular, magnocellular and possibly other inputs. The ventral stream, which is primarily concerned with perception, visual learning and object recognition, projects to the inferotemporal cortex; the dorsal projection stream, which controls action and prehension, projects to the posterior parietal lobe in association with the premotor and prefrontal areas (Servos, 2000).

Prehension (the action of taking hold) is a well-worked experimental model for fine motor control. Visually-guided prehension has two components: the *reach* (the kinetics of hand to object) and the *grasp* (influenced by object size, texture, composition, familiarity, distance, etc.). Prehension is not innate, and continues to mature for at least 9 years (Paré and Dugas, 1999). Central to the maturation of manual dexterity is the development of cortical motor-neural connections between the cortex and hand. Very young children make ineffective use of visual cues, so that acceleration and grasp force are not task-appropriate (i.e. a toddler is liable to crush a delicate object). After 4–5 years of age, children use their fast accumulating visual database and cognitive processes so that prehension can be anticipated and is more task-appropriate (Kuhtz-Buexchbeck *et al.*, 1999; Paré and Dugas, 1999). Children depend more on visual feedback than do adults during prehension (Kuhtz-Buexchbeck *et al.*, 1998).

Servos *et al.* (1992) have investigated the contribution of binocular vision to the accurate programming of prehensile movements. Monocular and binocular movements differed substantially. Under monocular viewing conditions, reaching latency was slower, velocity was lower; grasping was slower with smaller grip apertures, and subjects appeared to underestimate the distance of the objects. These authors proposed that binocularity contributes to the accurate programming of prehensile movements. More recently, Servos (2000) has suggested that monocular distance under-estimation in a prehension task has a visuomotor rather than a perceptual basis. In addition to this distance underestimation there is evidence that binocular vision is important for the calibration of the normal human grasp (Marotta *et al.*, 1997); however, when this information is not available the visuomotor system can use monocular cues, causing it to be more susceptible to pictorial illusions (Marotta *et al.*, 1998). Opinions differ over the role of binocular function in interceptive movements such as a catch. Bennett *et al.* (1999) provide evidence that binocular sources are important for this activity, which is not in accord with the findings of Servos and Goodale (1998). Gray and Regan (1998) and Bennett *et al.* (1999) conclude that prediction–motion tasks require both monocular and binocular information; but when objects are small, the former alone will not suffice (Gray and Regan, 1998).

AMBLYOPIA AND DISABILITY

Considering the tremendous scientific effort expended on understanding amblyopia and its clinical management, the lack of research on its functional impact is simply stunning and is a sad reflection of the level of interaction between basic and clinical science. There is ample experimental evidence that binocular function is important for a number of life's activities, especially fine hand–eye coordination. It is surprising that the fascinating studies on prehension, which have utilized normal subjects under binocular and monocular conditions, have not logically been extended to include individuals with amblyopia.

Of course, paucity of knowledge of functional impact of a medical condition is not unique to amblyopia and has a historical basis, perhaps because in the past there was a rather natural premise that any abnormality should be corrected, and evaluating functional significance was not a priority. Hence the statements in the introduction to this chapter by Snowdon and Stewart-Brown (1997) and Hartmann (1999), pointing out that the functional impact of amblyopia is unknown. So here I will touch on the evolving terminology of disability, and then attempt to review what is known about disability and amblyopia.

Classification of disability

The new International Classification of Functioning and Disability: ICIDH–2 (World Health Organization, 1999) covers any disturbance in terms of 'functional states' associated with health conditions – at body, individual and society levels. It employs terms that focus on the positive rather than negative aspects of functioning. Functioning and disability are umbrella terms covering three dimensions: body functions and structure (formerly impairment); activities at the individual level (formerly disability); and participation in society (formerly handicap). While the terms 'impairment' and 'disability' are still employed, the word 'handicap' is not (perhaps just as well considering its derivation: 'cap-in-hand').

ICIDH–2 only covers states that are associated with health conditions, i.e. it excludes socio-economic states. Impairments are bodily functions that deviate from the norm, while activity limitations (formerly disability) result when an individual has difficulty in performing an activity in an expected manner.

Loss of the better eye

The reported increased risk of individuals with amblyopia losing the fellow eye compared to ones without amblyopia (Tommila and Tarkkanen, 1981) is one of the most cited papers in grant applications for amblyopia research – presumably quoted to provide a *raison d'être* for the work proposed. An ocular disorder affecting individuals with amblyopia is more likely to affect the better eye more seriously than the one with amblyopia (von Leibiger, 1962; Vereecken and Brabant, 1984).

The concern that individuals with amblyopia are at risk of losing the fellow eye has been confirmed in a recent major UK-wide study of ophthalmologists by the British Ophthalmological Surveillance Unit (BOSU). Preliminary results from this study identified 257 adults with amblyopia who lost vision (from all causes) in the other eye within a 2-year period (Rahi *et al.*, 2000). Of these, 28 per cent were either blind or severely visually impaired (not defined), 26 per cent were unable to drive a motor vehicle, 15 per cent had more than one disability, and 44 per cent of those in paid employment were unable to continue. The annual age-specific incidence (per 100 000 total population in each age group) increased from 0.04 in children to 0.87 in those of 65 years or over. To date these findings have only been reported in abstract form; full publications are eagerly awaited.

However, a further observation that comes into play is the possibility of spontaneous visual improvement occurring in an amblyopic eye should the fellow eye be injured or succumb to disease. This phenomenon, though poorly quantified, is often manifest (see Moseley and Fielder, 2001, for a review). Indeed, some remarkable improvements (more than halving of letter acuity thresholds) have been reported (El Malleh *et al.*, 2000).

Implications for career

While we have already recognized that the functional implications of amblyopia are not well understood, certain occupations do require a high level of visual performance and defective vision in one eye precludes entry (Adams and Karas, 1999). These are mainly occupations involved with driving, navigating or piloting some form of moving vehicle, or the armed forces. Surprisingly these authors neglected to mention surgery, especially ophthalmic surgery, in which there is a widespread (but unsubstantiated) belief that binocular vision is important.

Refractive status, strabismus, amblyopia and disability

There is accumulated evidence (see Snowdon and Stewart-Brown, 1997 for a review of the impact of refractive error on disability) that defective (or absent) vision of one eye and strabismus may impact daily life. Although not clearly delineated, opinions do broadly concur that these three conditions are associated with the following disabilities: misjudging near and intermediate distances; reduced fine motor skills; clumsiness; somatization; interpersonal sensitivity; obsession–compulsion; and anxiety and depression. These are pertinent to education and occupation, lifestyle and sport.

However, hypermetropia, reduced monocular vision and strabismus are not independent variables, and may all be causally related depending on the circumstances. There is an urgent need therefore to undertake research on amblyopia and the disability that may occur, mindful of its ophthalmic and neurodevelopmental associations. It will also be interesting to learn whether any disability associated with amblyopia is related to the disruption of binocularity *per se*, or the level of vision, and whether the disabling effect is modified by adaptation throughout life.

If we fail to make progress in increasing our understanding of the disability associated with amblyopia, there is a danger that prioritized health service resources will be diverted to those areas where there is firmer evidence of a significant disability and effective treatment.

REFERENCES

Adams, G. G. W. and Karas, M. P. (1999). Effects of amblyopia on employment prospects. *Br. J. Ophthalmol.*, **83,** 380.

Alberman, E. D., Butler, N. R. and Gardiner, P. A. (1971). Children with squints: a handicapped child? *Practitioner*, **206,** 501–6.

Bauer, A., Kolling, G., Dietz, K. *et al.* (2000). Are cross-eyed persons worse drivers? The effect of stereoscopic disparity on driving skills. *Klin. Monatsbl. Augenheilk.*, **217,** 183–9.

Bax, M. and Whitmore, K. (1973). Neurodevelopmental screening in the school-entrant medical examination. *Lancet,* **ii,** 368–70.

Bennett, S., van der Kamp, J., Savelsbergh, G. J. P. and Davids, K. (1999) Timing a one-handed catch. I. Effects of telestereoscopic viewing. *Exp. Brain Res.*, **129,** 362–8.

Birch, E. E. (1993). Stereopsis in infants and its developmental relation to visual acuity. In: *Early Visual Development, Normal and Abnormal* (K. Simons, ed.), pp. 224–36. Oxford University Press.

Bishop, P. O. (1987). Binocular vision. In: *Adler's Physiology of the Eye: Clinical Application* (R. A. Moses and W. M. Hart, eds), pp. 619–89. C.V. Mosby Co.

Blake, R. and Fox, R. (1973). The psychophysical inquiry into binocular summation. *Percept. Psychophys.*, **14,** 161–85.

Brady, F. B. (1985). *A Singular View.* Brady.

Brown, M. M., Brown, G. C., Sharma, S. *et al.* (2001). Quality of life associated with unilateral and bilateral good vision. *Ophthalmol.*, **108,** 643–8.

Burden, A. L. (1994). The stigma of strabismus: an ophthalmologist's perspective. *Arch. Ophthalmol.*, **112,** 302.

Cartmill, M. (1992). Non-human primates. In: *The Cambridge Encyclopedia of Human Evolution* (S. Jones, R. Martin and D. Pilbeam, eds), pp. 24–32. Cambridge University Press.

El Mallah, M. K., Chakravarthy, U. and Hart, P. M. (2000). Amblyopia: is visual loss permanent? *Br. J. Ophthalmol.*, **84,** 952–6.

Fielder, A. R. and Moseley, M. J. (1996). Does stereopsis matter in humans? *Eye*, **10,** 233–8.

Godber, G. (1987). Living with one eye. *Br. Med. J.*, **295,** 1351.

Gray, R. and Regan, D. (1998). Accuracy of estimating time to collision using binocular and monocular information. *Vision Res.*, **38,** 400–512.

Hartmann, E. E. (1999). Brief overview of amblyopia. In: *Vision Screening in the Preschool Child* (E. E. Hartmann, ed.), pp. 16–19. National Maternal and Child Health Clearinghouse.

Heron, G., Dholakia, S., Collins, D. E. and McLaughlan, H. (1985). Stereoscopic threshold in children and adults. *Am. J. Optom. Physiol. Opt.*, **62,** 505–15.

Jeannerod, M., Arbib, M. A., Rizzolatti, G. and Sakata, H. (1995). Grasping objects: the cortical mechanisms of visuomotor transformation. *Trends Neurosci.*, **18,** 314–20.

Johnston, E. B., Cumming, B. G. and Parker, A. J. (1993). Integration of depth modules: stereopsis and texture. *Vision Res.*, **33,** 813–26.

Jones, R. K. and Lee, D. N. (1981). Why two eyes are better than one: the two views of binocular vision. *J. Exp. Psychol.*, **7,** 30–40.

Keltner, J. L. (1994). Strabismus surgery in adults. *Arch. Ophthalmol.*, **112,** 599–600.

Kuhtz-Buexchbeck, J. P., Stolze, H., Boczek-Funcke, A. B. *et al.* (1998). Kinematic analysis of prehension movements in children. *Behav. Brain Res.*, **93,** 131–41.

Kuhtz-Buexchbeck, J. P., Boczek-Funcke, A. B. and Illert, M. (1999). Prehension movement and motor development in children. *Exp. Brain Res.*, **128**, 65–8.

Kushner, B. J. (1994). Binocular field expansion in adults after surgery for esotropia. *Arch. Ophthalmol.*, **112**, 639–43.

Laidlaw, D. A., Harrad, R. A., Hopper, C. D. *et al.* (1998). Randomised trial of effectiveness of second eye cataract surgery. *Lancet*, **352**, 925–9.

Lemon, R. N. (1999). Neural control of dexterity: what has been achieved? *Exp. Brain Res.*, **128**, 6–12.

Marotta, J. J., Behrmann, M. and Goodale, M. A. (1997). The removal of binocular cues disrupts the calibration of grasping in patients with visual form agnosia. *Exp. Brain Res.*, **116**, 113–21.

Marotta, J. J., DeSouza, J. F. X, Haffenden, A. M. and Goodale, M. A. (1998). Does a monocularly presented size–contrast illusion influence grip aperture? *Neuropsychologica*, **36**, 491–7.

Milner, A. D. and Goodale, M. A. (1996). *The Visual Brain in Action.* Oxford Psychology Series No. 27.

Moseley, M. and Fielder, A. (2001). Improvement in amblyopic eye function and contralateral eye disease: evidence of residual plasticity. *Lancet*, **357**, 902–4.

Mruthyunjaya, P., Simon, J. W., Pickering, S. D. and Lininger, L. L. (1996). Subjective and objective outcomes of strabismus surgery in children. *J. Ped. Ophthalmol. Strab.*, **33**, 167–70.

Murdoch, J. R., McGhee, C. N. J. and Glover, V. (1991). The relationship between stereopsis and fine manual dexterity: pilot study of a new instrument. *Eye*, **5**, 642–3.

Packwood, E. A., Cruz, O. A., Rychwalski, P. J. and Keech, R. V. (1999). The psychosocial effects of amblyopia study. *J. Am. Assoc. Ped. Ophthalmol. Strab.*, **3**, 15–17.

Paré, M. and Dugas, C. (1999). Developmental changes in prehension during childhood. *Exp. Brain Res.*, **125**, 239–47.

Patterson, R. and Martin, W. L. (1992). Human stereopsis. *Human Factors*, **34**, 669–92.

Phillips, C. I. (1987). Personal view. *Br. Med. J.*, **295**, 1133.

Rahi, J. S., Logan, S., Timms, C. *et al.* (2000). Incidence and causes of new visual loss affecting the non-amblyopic eye of individuals with unilateral amblyopia in the United Kingdom. *Invest. Ophthalmol. Vis. Sci.*, **41**, S296.

Rogers, G. L, Chazan, S., Fellows, R. and Tsou, B. H. (1982). Strabismus surgery and its effect upon infant development in congenital esotropia. *Ophthalmology*, **89**, 479–83.

Satterfield, D., Keltner, J. L. and Morrison, T. L. (1993). Psychosocial aspects of strabismus study. *Arch. Ophthalmol.*, **111**, 1100–105.

Schor, C. (1991). Binocular sensory disorders. In: *Binocular Vision*, Vol. 9, *Vision and Visual Dysfunction* (D. Regan, ed.), pp. 179–223. Macmillan Press Scientific and Medical.

Servos, P. (2000). Distance estimation in the visual and visuomotor systems. *Exp. Brain Res.*, **130**, 35–47.

Servos, P. and Goodale, M. A. (1998). Monocular and binocular control of human interceptive movements. *Exp. Brain Res.*, **119**, 92–102.

Servos, P., Goodale, M. A. and Jakobson, L. S. (1992). The role of binocular vision in prehension, a kinetic analysis. *Vision Res.*, **32**, 1513–21.

Simons, K. (1981). Stereoacuity norms in young children. *Arch. Ophthalmol.*, **99**, 439–45.

Simons, K. (1993). Stereoscopic neurontropy and the origins of amblyopia and strabismus. In: *Early Visual Development, Normal and Abnormal* (K. Simons, ed.), pp. 409–53. Oxford University Press.

Snowdon, S. K. and Stewart-Brown, S. L. (1997). *Preschool Vision Screening: Results of a Systematic Review.* NHS Centre for Reviews and Dissemination.

Snyder, Q. S. and Lezotte, D. C. (1993). Prospective assessment of stereoscopic visual status and USAF pilot training attrition. *Aviat. Space Environ. Med.*, **64**, 14–19.

Stewart-Brown, S., Haslum, M. N. and Butler, N. (1985). Educational attainment of 10-year-old children with treated and untreated visual defects. *Dev. Med. Child Neurol.*, **27**, 504–13.

Stuart, G. W., Edwards, M. and Cook, M. L. (1992). Colour inputs to random-dot stereopsis. *Perception*, **21**, 717–29.

Tommila, V. and Tarkkanen, A. (1981). Incidence of loss of vision in the healthy eye in amblyopia. *Br. J. Ophthalmol.*, **65**, 575–7.

Vereecken, E. P. and Brabant, P. (1984). Prognosis for vision in amblyopia after the loss of the good eye. *Arch. Ophthalmol.*, **102**, 220–24.

von Leibiger, W. (1962) Über unterschiedliche Erkrankungshäufigkeit des amblyopen und des night ambyopen Auges. *Monatsbl. Augenheilk.*, **141**, 217–25.

von Noorden, G. K. (1990). *Binocular Vision and Ocular Motility. Theory and Management of Strabismus*, 4th ed. CV Mosby Co.

Wickens, C. D., Merwin, D. H. and Lin, E. L. (1994). Implications of graphics enhancements for the visualization of scientific data: dimensional integrality, stereopsis, motion and mesh. *Human Factors*, **36**, 44–61.

Westheimer, G. (1994). The Ferrier Lecture, 1992. Seeing depth with two eyes: stereopsis. *Proc. R. Soc. Lond. B*, **257**, 205–14.

Westlake, W. (2001). Is a one eyed racing driver safe to compete? Formula one (eye) or two? *Br. J. Ophthalmol.*, **85**, 619–24.

Wheeler, M. B., Stonesifer, K. and Kenny, M. (1979). Developmental evaluation in congenital esotropia. *Ophthalmology*, **86**, 2161–4.

World Health Organization (1999). *International Classification of Functioning and Disability.* ICIDH–2 Beta–2 draft.

Appendix

TRANSCRIPT OF *AMBLYOPIA: FROM TAXONOMY TO TREATMENT.*
A NOVARTIS FOUNDATION DISCUSSION MEETING HELD ON
20 JANUARY 1999, PORTLAND PLACE, LONDON

Organizers:
Merrick Moseley, Alistair Fielder, Gregory Bock (Novartis Foundation)

Speakers:
Stephen Anderson, Alistair Fielder, Robert Hess, Lynne Kiorpes, Merrick Moseley, Barnaby Reeves

Session moderators:
Maths Abrahamsson, Janette Atkinson, Colin Blakemore, Robert Doran, Kurt Simons, François Vital-Durand, Cathy Williams

Contributing discussants:
Stephen Anderson, Janette Atkinson, Colin Blakemore, Michael Clarke, Robert Doran, Alistair Fielder, Mark Hankins, Richard Harrad, Robert Hess, Lynne Kiorpes, Merrick Moseley, Jugnoo Rahi, Barnaby Reeves, Kurt Simons, Ruxandra Sireteanu, Sarah Stewart-Brown, François Vital-Durand, Cathy Williams, Geoffrey Woodruff

The following transcript is divided into six parts; each corresponds to the discussion that took place following a subject review presented by the authors of the preceding chapters.

Editors' note: However comprehensive and explanatory readers may have found the preceding chapters, they do not, and do not seek to, describe the motivations, pressures and driving controversies that hover in the background of this subject. These matters come to the forefront when scientists get together informally, and we believe are captured in the following discussions between a group of established workers in the field, some with quite different perspectives and priorities. Readers may also detect the occasional lighter note: wit, after all, is the natural accompaniment to wisdom!

Part I. Discussion following a review: *Sensory Processing in Experimental Amblyopia*, presented by Lynne Kiorpes

Fielder: Can you induce anisometropic amblyopia in monkeys with a more typically human refractive error rather than the −10 dioptres you used?

Kiorpes: Yes, you can. Earl Smith has shown, using a variety of lens powers, that you can get amblyopic deficits with lower power lenses. You don't have to use such a dramatic lens, but you are more likely to get amblyopia with the higher lens power. Also, I have a monkey in my lab that happened to have a naturally occurring 3.5 dioptre anisometropia and that animal developed amblyopia naturally.

Atkinson: With a −10D lens, do you know where they are accommodating?

Kiorpes: I don't. I haven't measured accommodation in these animals.

Hess: Could I just ask you about the encounter rate for recording neurons in the amblyopic cortex? Do you find it is harder to find cells, or is it the same sort of sampling found in normal cortex? It bears upon the issue of whether there are in fact less cells driven by the amblyopic eye in strabismus.

Kiorpes: We don't generally see a dearth of cells driven by the amblyopic eye in strabismus. We seem to find a pretty even balance and, for cells that are dominated by one or the other eye, they seem to end up at either end of the ocular dominance histogram (not in the binocular categories).

Blakemore: Isn't that a different result from the one you reported in the *Journal of Neuroscience*? (Kiorpes *et al.*, 1988). There you described a number of strabismic animals with very unbalanced ocular dominance distributions. Have you changed your views? Are these different animals?

Kiorpes: Those are the ones that I showed you, I should qualify what I said, you're right. If the strabismic animal has an extremely deep amblyopia – we had three animals that had 1–1.5 cycles per degree cut-off frequencies – those animals did show an ocular dominance shift. We found very few cells relatively speaking that can be driven by the amblyopic eye in those cases, and what I would say is that in the case of a very deep amblyopia you end up with something that is more like anisometropia or a monocular deprivation effect, but in terms of the middle-range strabismic amblyopias (which I have shown here) there does not seem to be any evidence for a loss of cells.

Blakemore: In those cases, was the strabismus always surgically induced?

Kiorpes: Yes.

Blakemore: And the surgery was done, if I remember correctly, at about 4 weeks of age?

Kiorpes: Yes, 3 to 4 weeks.

Blakemore: Given the variability in results, and the fact that some of your strabismic animals essentially looked like very briefly deprived monocularly deprived animals, in terms of their neuronal ocular dominance, their level of psychophysical amblyopia and the neuronal acuity losses in the cortex, is there any possibility that they *were*, in fact, briefly monocularly deprived after surgery, because of temporary closure of the lids or cloudiness of the cornea? François Vital-Durand and I have shown that as little as a couple of days of monocular deprivation, specifically around 4 weeks of age, induces similar effects on ocular dominance and so on, but we have never seen significant ocular dominance shifts in animals made strabismic at birth, when the system is much less sensitive to the effects of monocular deprivation.

Kiorpes: The three animals that have the very profound shift also had their strabismus created at 2 to 3 weeks. I don't believe that any of our surgically strabismic animals developed a ptosis. We have seen ptosis in the animals in which we created a strabismus with neurotoxin, but their visual behaviour is not necessarily more dramatically depressed than that of our surgically strabismic animals, so I can't say that it's a likely possibility. I think probably creating the strabismus earlier might have that effect more than necessarily looking for a monocular deprivation. What we also see is that some animals immediately adopt a unilateral fixation pattern very early and essentially never use the deviated eye. That could explain the difference, because two of those animals that we are talking about developed a unilateral fixation pattern very early, immediately after the surgery. Adopting a uniformly unilateral fixation pattern could create an effect like a monocular deprivation because the animal would be just suppressing the input from the other eye.

Anderson: Did you see any significant differences between the natural esotropes and the surgically induced esotropes?

Kiorpes: Not in terms of their visual behaviour. I have not recorded from any of the naturally strabismic animals. There are some data from them in the literature, but I've not done it myself. They tended to develop more moderate amblyopias than the ones we've done surgically so that the range of amblyopia that I saw in the naturally strabismic monkeys was a little smaller than that in the surgically strabismic, but then again there were many fewer naturally strabismic monkeys.

Atkinson: Can I ask a point of information about ocular dominance columns? I notice that yours for the normals looks very flat across 1–7, but the traditional ones I've seen for normals are more 'peaky' in the middle. Now, is that likely to be a significant difference? Because if you think about it, if you lost the peak in the middle, you might end up with something that looked rather different at the end.

Kiorpes: That's a difference, I think, between cats and monkeys. In cats you find a very peaky distribution – correct me if I am wrong – and much more binocular in that sense, whereas in monkeys most people find a much flatter distribution across the columns.

Blakemore: May I comment on that? The shape of the ocular dominance distribution in macaque monkeys depends very much on what fraction of neurons are sampled in layer 4c, because those cells are mainly monocular. If your microelectrode happens to spend a lot of time in 4c you can get huge numbers of monocular units and hence bias the overall distribution. Hubel and Wiesel's early ocular dominance histograms for the monkey were almost like those of strabismic cats, and I think that they were weighted towards layer 4c.

Harrad: Can I ask what happened to the naturally occurring strabismic monkeys? Did they 'get bullied in the playground?' Did they have any social interaction problems as a result of their strabismus?

Kiorpes: No! The naturally strabismic and the experimental strabismus monkeys did not get bullied by the others. Monkeys are very dominance-oriented animals, and the low dominance animal gets bullied no matter what it looks like for the most part. So no, I didn't see that those animals were ever at a particular disadvantage in the colony. What we did find though was that most of the naturally strabismic monkeys were rejected by their mothers so they ended up in the nursery – that's how we found them. That might be an interesting anecdotal point: that their mothers found something unusual about them, and these weren't necessarily mothers that normally rejected their offspring.

Simons: On the question of the applicability of the animal model to humans: you are all familiar with the argument . . . 'yes, but most of the animal model literature has been based on deprivation and so is not representative of the origin of most human amblyopia'. One related question I have never seen addressed is that a lot of the spatial performance data in animal studies has been based on gratings, which of course we know from the clinical literature are not a reliable measure of amblyopia. I'm wondering if to produce an amblyopia in an animal measurable with a grating test you have to exaggerate the degree of amblyopia? I was wondering why it is that no one in the monkey world has used something like a surrounded single-optotype tumbling E, which I would think you could train a monkey to do, to lay this whole question to rest.

Kiorpes: Von Noorden did it in his very early studies in the '70s.

Simons: But that was not surrounded, that was just a single optotype, which of course has the same deficit underestimation problem as the grating.

Kiorpes: It was a Landolt 'C', and I don't think he was very concerned about the issue of crowding. No one that I know has done in animals the equivalent of the crowded optotype test. However, what I would say is that I can show you the relationships between the deficits that our monkeys show on vernier and grating acuity as compared to comparably tested adult humans tested in the CACS study. Their measure of acuity was logMAR and they used a variety of different ways to measure it, including optotype acuity and grating acuity. The extent of the loss in vernier acuity is of the same order of magnitude in human and monkey strabismic amblyopes, which is related one-to-one, especially in anisometropic amblyopes, to the extent of the loss in Snellen acuity.

Woodruff: I notice that in your human data you have some mixed anisometropic and strabismic patients. I wonder whether monkeys with contact lens-induced anisometropia go on to develop strabismus, and how do they behave? How do they compare with the human anisostrabismic patients, who are not rare: they may represent 20 per cent of our patients with amblyopia, and they are certainly the most difficult to treat.

Kiorpes: Yes, a good question. Actually we do see mixtures, and what I've seen particularly in a lens-reared monkey is a large exotropia, which was surprising to me. But the exotropia did not develop during the rearing period; then, eye alignment was fine. So I don't think it affected his visual development *per se*. After the rearing period we took the lenses off and he became an exotrope. In several of the atropine-reared monkeys we saw some small strabismus. Now, what we've seen in the strabismic, and in the lens-reared monkeys, is that they sometimes develop a natural anisometropia which we think is related to their amblyopia. So it actually creates a kind of odd circular situation where the animals that developed amblyopia as a result of this rearing were more likely to develop an anisometropia naturally. This suggests that there is an interaction among these conditions between strabismus, amblyopia, and anisometropia that in the clinic may be very difficult to untangle. I've looked specifically at two monkeys who were made esotropic by surgical strabismus at around 3 to 4 weeks. We refracted them regularly as they were growing up. Both developed a natural anisometropia, one at around 10 weeks and the other one later, around 25 weeks. The anisometropia was always hypermetropia in the deviating eye.

Woodruff: You're saying that you have animals in whom you have surgically induced strabismus and they have subsequently developed anisometropia and that you have also seen monkeys in whom you have induced anisometropia and who subsequently developed strabismus. Is that correct?

Kiorpes: Yes.

Woodruff: That is very interesting for the clinicians because there is some debate as to which comes first. You seem to be saying that you have animal evidence that either can come first and either can be consequent to the other.

Kiorpes: That is what I am saying. I've seen it both ways around.

Sireteanu: In your surgical studies in monkeys you probably looked very early at their eye alignment. Do you see a consistent tendency of the initial deviation to be reduced, or to disappear, and how does this relate to their function afterwards?

Kiorpes: We don't necessarily. If the size of the deviation changes it does tend to get smaller, but we've seen them get larger as well. For the most part they seem to stay pretty much the same size. In the study that I showed you, the initial deviation was very closely correlated to the final deviation. We do not see any relationship between the size of the deviation itself and the visual outcome, but if you have an animal with an enormous squint it is more likely to develop amblyopia. All of the animals that had very large deviations developed amblyopia, but for smaller deviations there was no clear relationship between deviation size and amblyopia.

Sireteanu: Are the monkeys still amblyopic? Do you have microstrabismus in monkeys?

Kiorpes: I have never seen a deviation go completely away. It would instead become a small alternate strabismus. I can't easily measure microstrabismus, so I don't know if they have them. The amblyopic animals do maintain their amblyopia. I've not really seen the amblyopia go away in any of those animals.

Vital-Durand: I'm very puzzled by the facts still. I think there is a common law of development, proposed by Ron Boothe, which states that 1 week in monkeys is equivalent to 1 year in humans. Obviously, this is only a rough comparison. Adding that to individual differences could explain the variability of the magnitude of the deficits observed.

Kiorpes: I'm not sure how much I can satisfy your concerns. But I actually think it's a good thing that we see variability in monkey models because you see a huge range of variation in human populations in the outcome following strabismus and anisometropia. I think the fact that we have this much variation in the monkey means that we are accurately modelling the natural course of the disorder; it is a variable outcome disorder. I know that the variability in the strabismic animals has something to do with the fixation pattern the monkey adopts; those that alternate tend to avoid amblyopia. But what determines the fixation pattern they adopt, I don't know.

Part II. Discussion following a review: *Sensory Processing in Human Amblyopia*, presented by Robert Hess

Blakemore: The distinction that you draw between strabismic and non-strabismic amblyopia fits very well with the impression that Vital-Durand and I have gained from neurophysiological studies. In a substantial number of esotropic monkeys, in some of which we have demonstrated a clear deficit in acuity for gratings, we have never seen either a convincing shift in ocular dominance in the cortex or a convincing reduction in the spatial resolution of cortical neurons. We find that neurons driven through the strabismic eye have resolution within the normal range, some of them responding well to gratings of much higher spatial frequency than can be seen by the animal itself on a behavioural task. So I think we have to look beyond V1, or, as you were implying, at some subtle interactions in the coding between the elements in V1, to discover the primary deficit in strabismic amblyopia. Monocular deprivation and anisometropia, as Lynne has described, produce substantial changes in the resolution of individual neurons in V1, which presumably contribute to the amblyopia. However, even in these conditions, the loss of neuronal acuity in V1 is not sufficient to account for the entire behavioural deficit. The dramatic shift in ocular dominance that is also caused by deprivation or anisometropia might result in under-sampling of the image, which could also contribute to the amblyopia, but I suspect that there is also some additional component beyond V1, even in the case of this kind of amblyopia (which Vital-Durand and I refer to as 'blur' amblyopia, to distinguish it from strabismic amblyopia).

Hess: That's very interesting, it bears out my current prejudice that, at present, we do not have an adequate animal model of strabismic amblyopia in humans.

Sireteanu: We have data from cats, not monkeys, and the deficit seems to increase – there seems to be a cascade of increasing deficit as you go from striate to extrastriate areas. There is also a deficit in V1 which is not at the level of the single cells, but of the interaction between cells belonging to the amblyopic eye.

Sireteanu: You have mentioned the positional uncertainty but not the consistent positional error which sometimes also occurs in strabismic amblyopes, do you have data on this?

Hess: There isn't such a clear picture, let me just back up a little bit. In these types of measurements, where you are looking at the alignment of a central element you can measure two things: you can measure the accuracy with which you can tell the element is aligned and you can also measure the 50 per cent point, if you like, where the subject actually perceives the alignment to be. In cases of strabismic amblyopia it can be out of physical alignment, and that's what Ruxandra is referring to. We have looked at this in the same sort of detail, but we don't find the same sort of consistency. There can be large deficits that don't correlate with the accuracy deficits – they vary across the visual field in a different way, they don't necessarily scale with the accuracy deficit and we really don't know the origin of it. What we would like to do, and we've tried but unsuccessfully, is to do this experiment under perfectly stabilized conditions because then we would expect that if there is a distortion in the spatial representation, eye movements will not convert that into a loss of accuracy, accuracy should be perfect, you should just have an offset abnormality – a particular amblyope should see things misaligned but with normal accuracy.

Harrad: Robert, can I ask you a similar question? I was rather surprised to hear that positional uncertainty was constant across spatial scale, I would have thought that high spatial frequencies would be more affected in strabismics.

Hess: It's not an absolute, I mean there were cases where it was a little bit greater at the high scale and the line of best fit didn't really fit the data very well, but we looked at about 30 or so amblyopes and that's more the exception than the rule. The rule is – and certainly you never find any normal behaviour at low spatial frequencies – the abnormality is reasonably evenly distributed across spatial scale, but remember these stimuli we've used were adjusted for contrast so that they are all the same fraction above threshold for the amblyopic eye for the region of the visual field they're stimulated in, so we've factored out visibility. So some subjects won't be able to see the finer scale. That is one of the big differences between this measure of positional uncertainty and the vernier task. It is a task where just because the stimuli are sufficiently well separated from one another you have reduced the influence of local cues (i.e. contrast) so if you vary contrast it doesn't affect your performance in this three-element task whereas for the vernier task there is a strong dependence on contrast.

Kiorpes: Two things: one a comment and another a question about this same task. One of the slides I skipped over showed the physiology data from the periphery of one of our strabismic monkeys. It was interesting because that was the monkey that actually showed, in the foveal recordings, strong deficits in spatial resolution and contrast sensitivity for that population of cells. We went 15–20 degrees into the periphery in that animal to see if we saw a difference out there. In fact the distribution of cells in the periphery was perfectly matched between the amblyopic and the non-amblyopic eyes, so that the spatial deficit that we saw foveally in the cells was not there in the peripheral population.

Hess: So my prediction for the non-strabismic anisometropic animal is that if you did the same you would expect to find the same deficit for central and peripheral regions, if they have a behavioural deficit of course.

Kiorpes: We would expect to find it, yes, but we've not done that.

Hess: It's nice that you do the behaviour and the physiology because as you say there is such variation that you can't predict you're going to have the deficit.

Kiorpes: The question I had, I may have misunderstood your summary of the three-blob alignment task data, but it seemed as though there was a group of strabismics that actually sat at the bottom that looked very much like your non-strabismic subjects. There were also a number of strabismics that were off-scale, which are the ones that clearly show the positional uncertainty. I wonder if a) that is the right interpretation, and b) if there is some difference in the pool of strabismic amblyopes that would explain which ones look more like the non-strabismics on this task.

Hess: Well I don't think that is the correct interpretation overall, because all strabismics show significant positional deficits. These can range between a factor of 2 to 30. Anisometropes, even the most severe ones, never show as much as a factor of 2 loss in positional acuity once their contrast sensitivity abnormality has been accounted for. Obviously one would need more subjects to be able to know whether there are subgroups within either the strabismic or the non-strabismic camps. Our approach has been to do detailed measurements on a relatively small sample of amblyopes, typically around 20. There is a need for summary measures to be used on a larger population of amblyopes. I think only then could I really make any statement on whether different subgroups are present within this strabismic population for positional deficits.

Simons: Two questions: Are you familiar with the work that David Regan has done with his matrix acuity test suggesting a fixation control deficit basis for amblyopia versus a neural lateral interaction basis? You've mentioned the idea of using stabilized images. If Regan's conclusion has any validity that would be a critical experiment, to determine if there is in fact some kind of oculomotor component in the deficit, and not just in a simple image-smearing sense. My second question involves the comment I'm sure you've heard, that the central problem with all the positional uncertainty literature is that it's all based on adult amblyopes – i.e. a population of treatment failures. I am wondering if you can conceive of any possible way of obtaining a positional uncertainty measure for a test that could be used with a paediatric population. A 'before' and 'after' treatment measure in that age range would probably tell you a lot more about how generalizable these findings really are.

Hess: I think it is really important that we do that. In adults we certainly see similar results whether they had been treated or not, whether surgically or by orthoptic treatment. We have to begin to do this with children, and it can certainly be done.

Simons: But you would have to have a new test format.

Hess: Yes, using a completely new test format, but it can be done for a detection task where you compare three elements that are aligned with three elements in which one is misaligned – telling the odd one out – and we have some pilot data. It would be nice to know what happens in visual development, and my initial thought about this positional alignment is that it is really a bottom-up sort of process but I'm also beginning to believe more and more that there are quite big top-down influences, that it really could involve a lot of processing from extrastriate areas. As I have said before, vernier acuity, with its strong dependence on contrast, is a very different type of positional measure to the one I have discussed today. Our knowledge of how positional sensitivity changes in early visual development has been exclusively based on vernier acuity measurements, and I don't think that this bears upon the issue I am discussing today.

Sireteanu: My colleague Maria Fronius is collecting the data that you suggest. She has produced a simple paediatric version of the test able to measure positional error and positional uncertainty. She is studying children undergoing treatment and those yet to be treated by patching and vision therapy.

Hess: Is it too early to say what the outcome is?

Sireteanu: Positional uncertainty is reduced at the same time as acuity improves, practically hand-in-hand. But positional error has a different dynamic, sometimes under occlusion of the other eye it might become even worse and then it stabilizes at some point. So the two of them do not seem to be related, they seem to have different substrates.

Hess: Interesting, it bears out my finding that contrast sensitivity and positional losses are quite independent.

Fielder: In appraising disability we have to think about what people see with both their eyes open. Is there a visual deficit in amblyopic individuals when they have both eyes open?

Hess: Well this relates to whether their normal eye is really normal. In a lot of the studies we typically use the normal eye as a control because it's so convenient – we factor out individual variability and we don't have to do normal populations. In general it *is* normal, but there are plenty of documented cases where one can pick up slight differences between the fellow eye of an amblyope and a normal eye of a non-amblyopic observer; not in an absolute sensitivity but usually in how that sensitivity varies across different parameters such as contrast sensitivity, spatial alignment, temporal sensitivity. These are relatively subtle differences, but although they may be quite important for the individual, I don't think they are important insofar as your question is directed towards disability. I think that the vision they have through their normal eye is essentially normal and they are really not disadvantaged to a great extent in having an amblyopic eye except in terms of stereopsis and so forth, which some people think is very important and some people think is rather unimportant. We should not underestimate the importance of having two normal eyes in case one is lost later in life.

Moseley: Those of us who have submitted grant applications for peer review in order to fund investigations of treatment evaluation often receive criticism when we say we intend to measure (just) acuity and/or contrast sensitivity. We get critical feedback suggesting dozens of other tasks we could be measuring. Our general riposte is that such a reviewer is simply not familiar with what you can and what you can't do with $3\frac{1}{2}$-year-old children. But given that, should we be looking at positional uncertainty as a treatment outcome? Are there any such tests available on the horizon?

Hess: Can I just make a plea, that is if anyone comes up with a test of positional uncertainty make sure that it doesn't depend very much on contrast. Otherwise you are always going to be up against the criticism 'well, doesn't that just follow as a consequence of the contrast sensitivity loss?'. So you need one that is relatively insensitive to contrast, but I think it is inappropriate to use it just yet because firstly we haven't really developed it sufficiently for this population and secondly it could get a bad press if it's used inappropriately early on. It would be good for just one or two places to do this work, adopting an experimental approach. Remember that it has been 10 or 15 years since we've known about this, and it still hasn't trickled down to the clinic.

Harrad: I know that Ilona Kovacs designed a test of looking for little Gabors that's a similar sort of positional task, is it not?

Hess: The test to which you allude was not designed to measure positional uncertainty but contour integration.

Harrad: Can you elaborate?

Hess: David Field, William McIlhagga and myself have shown that amblyopes are abnormal on contour integration tasks of this kind, but it has in fact nothing to do with contour integration *per se*. Amblyopes have positional uncertainty, and this limits their ability to integrate contours. We showed that if you measure the positional uncertainty in the amblyopic eye and incorporate that into the contour integration stimulus for the normal eye, then this mimics the amblyopes's performance on a contour integration task. This implies that it is positional uncertainty, not contour integration, that is abnormal in amblyopia. I think it would be simpler to measure positional uncertainty directly rather than its indirect effects on contour integration. The three-element alignment task that I described should be an ideal way of doing it with children.

Fielder: Can I just pick up on what you said about 'trickling down to the clinic'? There is also the problem of 'creeping up to the lab', because that information about failure of emmetropization in strabismus has been known in the clinical world for two decades or so.

Part III. Discussion following a review: *Functional Imaging in Amblyopia*, presented by Stephen Anderson

Atkinson: Can I open the discussion by asking if your stimulus is really picking up more than just a contrast decrease in the amblyopic eye because you use quite low contrast red–green stimuli?

Anderson: No, the stimuli were not low contrast. They were physically isoluminant patterns with a contrast of 80–90 per cent.

Atkinson: But don't you think that the difference in the extent above psychophysical threshold matters for the amblyopic eyes?

Anderson: Not at the spatial frequencies we're dealing with, no.

Hess: Stephen, it is curious that you don't get very good responses to low spatial frequencies where at least the chromatic signal is at its best. Surely there is a brain region not too far away that must be responding to that?

Anderson: Well, there are two factors here. Firstly, MEG is sensitive to the number of cycles in the display and as we had a long viewing distance our low spatial frequency patterns were necessarily limited in size. Therefore, at least some of the decline in magnetic field power at low frequencies is probably due to the restricted number of cycles displayed. However, I don't think that's the main reason why the MEG and psychophysical measures differ as they do. I don't have an answer for it, except to say that I am never surprised by huge differences between functional imaging studies and psychophysics; they are measuring entirely different things. The amplitude of the MEG responses reflects the number of active neurones and, importantly, the extent to which they are synchronously active. The CSF, on the other hand, reflects the performance limit of the visual system as a whole, and there is some evidence that this limit may be based on the activity of a relatively small number of neurones. Sensitivity at low spatial frequencies might, for example, be determined by a small number of units – perhaps too small to be recorded with MEG. As the receptive fields of low spatial frequency units are larger, fewer of them are needed for effective sampling, but their large fields would make them very sensitive.

Hess: But it might follow then, as a consequence, that if you reduce the contrast of your stimulus and become closer to where some of us believe the contrast sensitivity abnormality is, that the curves might separate even more.

Anderson: We have played around with contrast, but not specifically to look at that.

Blakemore: If you are arguing that an early cortical defect (in V1 or perhaps V2) underlies amblyopia, it would be good to see some quantitative relationship between MEG signals and the depth of amblyopia. However, you said that you didn't see a correlation with Snellen acuity. In a study of visual evoked potentials (VEPs) in which I was involved (Kubova *et al.*, 1996) we *did* see a clear correlation for responses from the occipital pole, which was especially clear at high spatial frequencies. Now, I saw that your responses were cutting off at 2–4 c/deg – a region of the spatial frequency spectrum in which most amblyopes don't have a deficit anyway.

Anderson: But remember we used red–green modulated stimuli positioned in the peripheral retina. If you compare the psychophysical acuity limit for the part of the retina we examined, it is not far removed from our MEG measures. The extrapolated acuity limit based on contrast sensitivity measures for our stimulus is only about 8–9 c/deg.

Blakemore: Well in that case it would be useful to see a comparison between your MEG results and psychophysical performance for exactly the same stimulus in the same part of the visual field, rather than a comparison with Snellen acuity in central vision.

Anderson: Yes. I didn't have time to show those results, but I have measured the chromatic CSF under identical laboratory conditions. The estimated acuity is a bit higher with contrast sensitivity measures and, as Robert said, the CSF is low pass whereas the MEG tuning curve is band pass. I think that these differences arise because the psychophysical limit reflects the activity of a few number of units; and MEG simply isn't sensitive enough to record activity from a small number of neurones. Knowing that you would be here, and with the Kubova paper in mind, I did think about the relationship you found between VEP amplitude and Snellen acuity. There is of course considerable individual variability in the amplitude of responses obtained with both VEPs and MEG. We only examined six amblyopes, so it is possible that we may have found a correlation with acuity had we examined more subjects. I don't know.

Stewart-Brown: Can I ask you a question from an epidemiological perspective that may turn out to be rather naïve? It seems to me that you've demonstrated that there are some abnormalities or differences in the visual cortex in a small number of people who also have amblyopia, and that these abnormalities may be associated with one another. However, I am getting the impression from what you are saying that you believe there to be a causal relationship. In epidemiology we would have to do quite a lot more to show that if A and B are associated with each other, that one was causing the other, rather than that they were occurring together for other reasons, or that the amblyopia caused the abnormality in the brain. I just wonder if you could enlighten me about the sort of steps you take in your field.

Anderson: Well I'm always nervous when someone begins by saying this may be a naïve question! I'll try my best, but I'm not quite sure what causal relationship you are getting at here; these are amblyopes and they have a cortical deficit.

Stewart-Brown: But they could occur together for some unrelated reason, or the cortical deficit could occur secondary to the amblyopia because having amblyopia in childhood might result in a different development of the visual cortex so you pick up this abnormality in adults. How can you go from what you have demonstrated to being clearer about the belief that it is the cause of amblyopia?

Hess: Let me give a possible example. If, say, the geometry of the cortex was slightly changed in a particular subject but visual function was normal, one might obtain differences in the MEG response.

Fielder: This is absolutely fundamental to medical practice because you get so many events occurring at the same time. To pick up on Geoffrey Woodruff's comment, you may have a strabismic who may have been anisometropic in the first place. Which came first, the cart or the horse?

Stewart-Brown: I suppose it comes back to my again very outsider's belief, that the infant brain is pretty plastic and there are all sorts of stuff about the development of the brain and the human infant that we are not very clear about and that you can develop different pathways depending on where you happen to be and what your environment is and what seems to make sense to your brain at that time.

Atkinson: (to Anderson) I think you are quite right in pointing out that this is a fundamental correlation and you can presumably do some tests, even MEG tests on the amblyopic eye and the non-amblyopic eye showing that there was absolutely no difference between the two eyes' responses, but that there were also cortical responses in some other area. That would, in a way, limit you to saying that this correlation was possibly specific to a domain and not across domains. It wouldn't however give you any handle on the causal events, and I don't think you are ever expecting to get a handle on the causal events here. All you are really trying to do is to point out the fundamental mechanisms that might have gone astray as a result of the early deficit.

Blakemore: Jan, if there were no neurons in the brain that could respond to a particular visual stimulus, then there would surely be no possibility that the animal or person could see such a stimulus. So, that would surely imply a causal relationship between neuronal activity (or inactivity) and behaviour. The studies of neuronal activity in animals help to reinforce the link between human psychophysics and studies of human MEG and VEP. When a monkey is monocularly deprived, there is a gradual erosion in the ability of neurons in the primary visual cortex to resolve gratings, which surely sets a limit on what the animal will be able to detect.

Fielder: I'm slightly confused. Do you mean that there is a progressive deterioration, or a failure to develop?

Blakemore: Both. It depends how prolonged the deprivation is. In normal monkeys, the spatial resolution of neurons in V1 (just as in the lateral geniculate nucleus) increases substantially and gradually over the first few months of life. We think that this process is, to a large extent, a passive reflection of the increasing angular density of central retinal cones, as the eyeball grows and the foveal cones become more tightly packed (Jacobs and Blakemore, 1988). For relatively short periods of monocular deprivation, the rate of improvement of resolution of neurons driven through the deprived eye is simply slowed, but if deprivation is prolonged (beyond a few weeks, at the height of the sensitive period), then there is a real decrease in performance, below that seen shortly after birth (when the best cells can resolve about 1 c/deg). Of course, if the normal maturation is largely passive, any decrease in the rate of improvement is likely to reflect some *active* process of degradation caused by deprivation.

Stewart-Brown: Isn't that an experimental situation in which you are showing artificially induced amblyopia can lead to these changes in the brain? I am talking about a naturally occurring condition which might also subsequently give rise to these problems in the brain, and the naturally occurring condition might have another cause.

Kiorpes: If you have a naturally occurring strabismus, whether it is in the human or monkey, you can actually expect a certain effect on the time course of visual development for that strabismic person or monkey, and I think those things can be concluded to be relatively causal. I don't see that it is much of a stretch to go from looking at the development of a monkey strabismic versus a human strabismic. Is that the point you're making? Because I think that what some of our studies have shown, more than the studies of others, is that the kind of amblyopia that you see in monkeys, whether they are naturally strabismic or surgically strabismic, is basically the same, and that it is very similar to what you see in human adult strabismic amblyopes. So I think it is reasonable to deduce from the data of a developing strabismic animal what you might expect to find developing in a human strabismic.

Simons: Just to underline the point . . . there *are* naturally strabismic monkeys . . .

Hankins: One presumes that because of the nature of your technique you are sampling quite superficially?

Anderson: Yes, it's only limited to shallow sources, especially as a second-order gradiometer was used.

Hankins: So that presumes that your signal is dominated by more binocularly driven signals. Does that in some way impinge on the difference you might see with VEP?

Anderson: No, I don't believe so. I think many of the differences between VEPs and MEG relate to the fact that VEPs are much more sensitive to far-field sources and because electrical measures, unlike magnetic measures, are distorted by volume conductance through the head.

Can I just go back slightly to the question before . . . the problem we have, if I'm picking up on you correctly, is that we cannot know the extent to which the deficits we measure are simply developmental artefacts. Is that what you are saying?

Stewart-Brown: . . . or possibly associated with it, but not fundamental.

Atkinson: There is a fundamental point here, which is that if, say, your MEG result had been obtained from a child with amblyopia who also had cerebral palsy, we would not have made the same assumptions about the causal relationships. We would have said that there was a fundamental difference in this child's brain compared to normals. What Sarah is saying is, if there is such a high incidence of visual anomaly and strabismus in clinical populations, how can we be sure that we're not just picking up, with normal amblyopes, the tip of the iceberg? A particular measure might be brain functioning, cortex functioning at all different levels, and it may be just that the sensitivity of our technique is either too sensitive or less sensitive than it need be. Now that is putting it in a very gross way, but you can see how from the outsider's point of view there is a genuine argument about causality, and that is why it is fundamental to point out the normal responses of the amblyopic eye, in some other sense, to actually contrast the difference.

Anderson: Yes, I agree. Indeed, we show that the responses driven by the normal eye of amblyopes are similar to those evoked in non-amblyopic subjects. Also, in other areas of the brain, such as V5, we have not found any differences between the normal and amblyopic eye responses – though I should add that those experiments on V5 are not yet completed.

Sireteanu: You have said that if you have reduced amplitude you have prolonged latency, I guess you also have tuning curves for the latencies, so does development in latency depend on spatial frequency?

Anderson: No, I think the change in latency was approximately independent of spatial frequency – though I confess I have not looked closely at that.

Fielder: There have been a number of observations in which there are certain groups of children where the incidence of strabismus goes up to 30 or 50 per cent, and those are children who are born pre-term who have had particular eye diseases or neurological insults, and if you look at huge populations, and you look at their general behaviour (and again a lot of this stuff is pretty anecdotal but nevertheless relates to big populations of a thousand or so children), the children who have strabismus are actually clumsier than others. I'm just watching and seeing. In a way there is such a huge discrepancy between what we see in clinical life and what we see in the textbooks, and I see that discrepancy as terribly disturbing.

Clarke: As a clinician I think that it is very applicable to, for example, the situation of a monocular cataract in a child – the situation is a bit different and possibly more complex in an older child who becomes amblyopic at the age of 3 or 4, whereas the work that has been done might not be applicable to the state of the development of the nervous system in that child. I think that is perhaps one of the difficulties in clinical practice. Also, the interventions that are used in animal work are different from the pathologies that we see clinically in these older children where there are perhaps milder degrees of deprivation or blur or strabismus, which may actually have different outcomes and different mechanisms.

Woodruff: (to Anderson) Obviously I feel that all this neurophysiology has something to do with the patients I see in the clinic, but I have some sympathy for what Sarah [Stewart-Brown] is saying, particularly when I come across exceptions. You describe new psychophysical work with 'these results' and 'these subjects', and then there are a few subjects which did not fit with your thesis. Now some of the variations in your results are extremely interesting, and I am interested to know whether you think the variations are due to measurement variation – which we could all understand – or to what extent they are due to your different subjects having different kinds of amblyopia. Earlier we heard from Robert that if he could change his life, he'd have more subjects. I wonder whether the top of your wish list shouldn't be more information about the previous ophthalmic history of your subjects. Certainly as a clinician, I feel we don't know as much about these subjects as we'd like to.

Anderson: There is enormous variability when you look at the animal work in single-cell physiology, and I wonder – the physiologists may tear me down – but I wonder if some or all of that variability is due to sampling problems. You are really only measuring from a relatively few number of cells. The imaging work, on the other hand, reflects the activity of millions of cells in a given area, and probably the interactions between close areas. Because of this, MEG is sensitive to variations in cortical anatomy. I don't think the individual differences we find are due to different types of amblyopia within a group. I think that most of the individual variations we see come about because of the enormous variability in the size, location and sulcal pattern of the primary visual area. It is so variable that I no longer trust brain-imaging studies that rely on group averages to enhance their signal-to-noise levels. We did in fact test eight amblyopes and seven normals in this study. In two amblyopes and one normal we failed to obtain any occipital responses despite the fact that the MEG detectors were placed over the occipital cortex. This may have been because the architecture of their primary visual cortex rendered the evoked currents silent to MEG measures.

Kiorpes: I do have to point out that there is a huge range of variability for humans with a given condition: anisometropic amblyopia, strabismic amblyopia, and strabismus and anisometropia combined. These are adults that have grown up with whatever treatment history or non-treatment history they had, but nevertheless they are all amblyopes of a class. There is a huge range of variability in their deficits, and what psychophysicists and neurophysiologists and people who have tried to model these conditions try to do is to take specific sets of conditions that are known and say: what's the result of this amblyopiogenic condition under these known developmental conditions? What we can say about vision and visual performance in animals – and you still get a wide range of variability even under those very specific conditions – is, yes, there *is* a lot variability across individual brains with exactly the same conditions and there *is* going to be a lot of variability across kids, but what I would hope you would get from these kind of studies is that there is a very close correlation between what you see in animal models of amblyopia and what you see in the human population. You can then look at those psychophysical data and try to make some conclusions about what the important things are that you need to know about in terms of the mechanisms underlying visual development. It probably doesn't matter to the clinician whether this is a V1 or a V2 deficit in that very specific sense; what matters more to the clinician is that there is a change in the brain, and whether the change is fixable.

Anderson: I agree that there is considerable variability between patients, but I state again that I don't believe the individual differences we find with MEG reflect different possible subclasses of amblyopic patient. I would like to end by saying that I think it is important to determine the site of the amblyopic deficit so that any future drug and/or psychophysical treatments may be targeted to dysfunctional areas.

Simons: One key point underlying what Lynne was saying . . . the clinicians can't throw too many rocks at the neurophysiologists. Clinicians, as you are all very well aware, have their own classification nightmares – look at the battle over infantile esotropia's definition. Amblyopia is very difficult to define clinically (e.g. specifying its presence or deficit level on the basis of clinical chart vs. newspaper text reading), and so in some respects it is tidier in the neurophysiology literature.

Woodruff: I just want to say that with the monkey data that behaves differently from what you expect you should treasure the exceptions.

Part IV. Discussion following a review: *Taxonomy and Epidemiology of Amblyopia*, presented by Barnaby Reeves

Vital-Durand: I am very puzzled by the way you tend to question the ability and competence of your colleagues in the clinic. Is this a problem in this country?! You have just said that we have to be straightforward! Am I blind to what is happening in my own country? I have the feeling that by 6 months of age nobody should miss a microtropia. Would people agree with that?

Audience exclaims: No!

Vital-Durand: . . . by 7 months?

Atkinson: This is a case of French confidence in their ophthalmologists!

Clarke: Certainly when we looked at our screening data we found children at outcome who had microtropias who hadn't been diagnosed with having a microtropia when they were screened at 3 years and treated. It became apparent in the course of their treatment that they had a microtropia; whether that microtropia came on during the course of their treatment or whether it was there at 3 and was missed we couldn't determine, but my feeling is that you can miss microtropias, particularly in toddlers.

Atkinson: It is not any easier at 3 months or 5 months or even 6 months.

Vital-Durand: At 9 months, I would say it is possible.

Woodruff: In our study, some of our centres never diagnosed microtropia and some centres diagnosed it much more frequently.

Vital-Durand: Of course you will always miss 1 in 1000 . . .

Woodruff: This is a whole centre seeing 100 patients and they didn't see one, and another centre saw twelve.

Simons: One difficulty is that a lot of people use the 4-dioptre base-out prism, which is not a reliable test. There are atypical responses, so irrespective of the skill of the ophthalmologist in different countries, there is the question of the test's reliability to begin with. Microtropia is a little bit difficult to test for even with a co-operative older child. Second, I still think it is fair to say – and this is within countries and not simply between – that all studies are not created equal. One thing that bothers me about these summary run-downs of hundreds of studies is – to pick one example that Jan [Atkinson] is more familiar with than she would like to be – even paediatric ophthalmologists and certainly general ophthalmologists are definitely not all created equal in their ability to do retinoscopy. If you have a study that is making statements about astigmatism for instance, you have got to be careful to establish that its examiners adequately monitored where the child was fixating. I should mention, as an aside, that in the US we are about to start a large RCT that I think would fit all your requirements, comparing penalization with patching, and they are going to use paediatric ophthalmologists with strict quality control of data. I think that there is such an enormous amount of noise in the data we are concerned with that it is difficult to draw any serious conclusions about incidence in the first place. We've been attempting in the US to get a major study funded by the NEI simply to determine prevalence. The amblyopia epidemiology folks say you can't believe the extant statistics out there, despite the fact that there are probably a hundred studies, or close to it. Microtropia is just sort of the tip of the iceberg as far as the problems of mensuration. Moving on from that, you often don't have a reliable acuity measure, as most of these studies did not use a surrounded optotype. It goes on and on. I think the whole taxonomic question gets almost completely subverted by this mensuration problem, and until you get this latter problem sorted out you've just got to be real careful about making statements about the taxonomy.

Reeves: I don't disagree at all.

Atkinson: I think that the fundamental problem is that I agree with almost everything that you (Reeves) said. That's a problem in itself! But also for the natural history of amblyopia. We suspect that it occurs to some extent in some children in the first 3 years of life. We do not have a sensitive measure of amblyopia – possibly we do have a reliable measure of manifest strabismus, but even deciding whether they are an alternator or not an alternator would cause a fight in this room! We could probably measure and identify manifest strabismus in the first 3 years, but anything else we could not possibly measure properly, so we can't get the natural history of amblyopia. Kurt's very good study is starting with them at 4 years; we don't know what happened to them at 2 years. So if they are amblyopic at 4 years, we don't know what happened at 6 months or 9 months or at 2 or 3 years. We only know what they are at 4 years.

Simons: Can I also mention that I have, in press, in the *British Journal of Ophthalmology* (Simons and Preslan, 1999), an analysis demonstrating that there is in fact a good deal of evidence out there on natural history? For example, Mark Preslan's studies of an inner-city elementary school where it turned out that of all the children he detected having amblyopia in the first of his two studies (which were a year apart), not one of them was ever treated at all. So by default he had a natural history group, and it turns out there are several other studies out there totalling up to something like 1200 kids. So, as you would expect – and as you clinicians will all be relieved to know(!) – non-treatment of amblyopia does result in deterioration; there was no case of spontaneous improvement.

Reeves: Workshops of this kind are always valuable in bringing together people with different perspectives, but I wonder whether our perspectives are too different to broker agreement. I don't think even the most applied public health professionals among us would deny that the brain is plastic, and that it therefore almost certainly follows the same sort of developmental 'rules' that a monkey's or cat's brain follows. However, our different perspectives make us interested in different problems and ask different research questions. Neurophysiologists study amblyopia because they want to find out how the brain develops; public health doctors are interested in amblyopia in order to make difficult decisions about providing health care. If Jan's view is correct, that we cannot detect, treat and monitor children at a reasonable cost and with reasonable accuracy and efficiency between 6 months and 3 years when treatment is most likely to be effective, then the public health perspective becomes important.

Atkinson: I think the question we can answer at present is to take an older group and screen them properly and see whether treatment is effective at that stage. We could do this immediately as a first step.

Fielder: I don't think you would learn enough from that.

Atkinson: Why not?

Fielder: Well, you don't know the compliance.

Stewart-Brown: Barney, I thought that the studies you propose are very interesting and would be well worth doing, but I still don't think that they will answer the question, which is: is all this animal work which suggests that something is quite likely to work in humans actually valid? If the pharmaceutical industry, for example, had developed a drug in animals which appeared to be very effective and they just marketed it to the general population without first testing it in a well-controlled trial, they would be taken to the cleaners. It is just inconceivable that they could do that. Now we've reached this situation for very good reasons, we're doing something on the basis of animal studies that isn't validated in children, and I don't think that there is any way to address that other than doing a trial.

Reeves: I don't think that is historically true. Occlusion therapy started long before we had any neurophysiological evidence. Thousands of medical treatments have become established just because they work, without evaluation, and are still used without evaluation even now.

Stewart-Brown: An awful lot of those are now being evaluated where there is any question . . .

Reeves: Well, some of them are. However, carrying out a trial of occlusion therapy will not necessarily answer your question, because occlusion is not like a pharmaceutical treatment. For example, I am not convinced that it is possible to find a plausible placebo intervention to compare with occlusion or to mask the measurement of either beneficial or harmful outcomes. If one observes a small, non-significant difference given a sample size chosen in order to be able to detect a clinically important overall effect, the result is ambiguous given the kinds of other evidence that I have described.

Stewart-Brown: You will get an answer which is a great deal better than what we have now. It may not be perfect, no single trial is perfect, but if you do several different trials you will get an idea, and if you are getting a result that is not significant in the entire population but is in one subgroup then that is a very important difference that you shouldn't be missing. That would mean that there are a whole lot of children that are currently being treated at the moment whom you are doing either no good to or harming. Yes, it would be legitimate to test subgroups later on to see whether there was an effect. But you would stop applying treatment across the board on the basis that it might be helping a few of the children you were treating because treatment is not without its consequences.

Reeves: Well I think we have to agree to disagree.

Simons: It is historically important to see this whole animal issue in perspective. The animal folks came into the game late. Amblyopes have been treated by patching for at least 200 years, and von Noorden has dug up some manuscripts suggesting it goes back to the fourteenth century.

Harrad: Not peer reviewed . . .?!

Simons: That's right!

Doran: Does the problem get easier if you make the criteria for the diagnosis of amblyopia more difficult – i.e. you don't accept any amblyopia where the interocular acuity differs by less than 1 octave, and you don't accept any clinical observation in the records you are reviewing unless it is repeated. The thing about clinical work is that you observe, then you observe again, and then observe again so that variations can be ironed out.

Reeves: I think the problem certainly does get easier if you do. That is why I say we need to do these large prospective, longitudinal cohort studies with careful clinical evaluations where the data are collected systematically and according to agreed definitions. Such studies are very difficult to do, arguably as difficult as large randomized trials. Where Sarah and I disagree, I think, is that I would rather do a cohort study first and try to get more evidence about the precise research questions we should be asking before starting a randomized controlled trial. At the very least, I think we should be doing both kinds of study side-by-side.

Doran: I was present at a fascinating meeting at Mike Clarke's department in Newcastle, where we were being educated as to the raw requirements for such an epidemiological exercise, and there was some feeling there that we ought not to include amblyopes who had severe amblyopia – i.e. worse than 6/24. I would argue strongly that they *should* be included, because I have no embarrassment about the potential for treatment at the right time based on the perceived severity of the amblyopia.

Clarke: I think one of the differences between a screening programme and ordinary medical treatment is that we are offering a programme which requires that we should have a greater knowledge of the natural history and of treatment effects than for the situation where a parent comes to us saying, 'my child doesn't see well out of one eye, can you help, doctor?'.

Reeves: In principle, I agree. However, the detection of amblyopia is rather different since the disease is 'asymptomatic' primarily because the patient is a young child – a $3\frac{1}{2}$-year-old child with anisometropia isn't going to come up to you and say 'doctor, doctor, I can't see out of one eye'. If an amblyopic child is detected by case finding with a clinically important reduction in visual acuity, I suggest that there would be little clinical uncertainty about the need to monitor the child and treat the amblyopia.

Fielder: If you were setting up a screening programme today, then I accept Mike's point, but when screening was set up 20 years ago the assumption was just to help people.

Clarke: There are clear criteria now, and we are also more aware of the downside of screening. I'm not criticizing people who introduced screening, I'm just saying that we have arrived at a point where if we are going to continue offering a screening programme we need a better level of evidence.

Reeves: There is a pragmatic, cost-effectiveness issue here, quite apart from whether screening and treatment for amblyopia works. If comprehensive NHS screening is stopped, private optometrists will offer screening. In the UK, where the cost of private eye tests for children is reimbursed by the NHS, this will be much more expensive, and less effective. Moreover, the NHS will be paying for children to be tested more than once because of the financial incentive for optometrists to recall children for an examination.

Clarke: I agree with that absolutely, but I think unless there is a better level of evidence screening programmes will start to go, and have already started to go in some areas of the country.

Reeves: If some Health Authorities are stopping screening, then we really ought to be setting up the epidemiological studies to compare the visual outcomes for children in Health Authorities that do screening with health authorities that do not.

Simons: One thing from somebody from outside the country who doesn't understand NHS politics at all, but which absolutely stands up like a billboard to me, is that we have sitting in the middle of this room a no-longer so young lady with some grey hair named Jan Atkinson who has undertaken – there's a good reason for my comment Jan, I didn't just say that for nothing! – who has undertaken to my mind one of the most important studies in the history of this specialty, looking at a far more dramatic issue than the effect of treatment. She's been looking at prophylaxis as nobody has done before. The reason for the grey hair remark, Jan, is that you might say she got that from attempting the huge task of doing a major study of this matter! I don't want to make charges about hypocrisy, and I'm aware that political systems are complicated in every country, but I do find it more than a little ironic that there's all these rocks being thrown at screening while at the same time here's Jan's study, done prospectively, set up as close to ideal as possible, and demonstrating in an unprecedented way the utility of (early) screening!

Atkinson: But there are a lot of other people in this room who are attempting to do the same thing . . . Cathy Williams over there is one.

Simons: No grey hair, I couldn't tell!

Atkinson: But she, she's younger than me! She's been doing it less years – a few less years, but this is precisely why I say at the moment I think it is very difficult to get the true natural history of amblyopia. We have been trying for 15 years to get good measurement of early amblyopia, and I would say that that is one of the weakest parts of our follow-up study. The secondary part is not so much the screening programme, but there is absolutely no point in devising very good screening programmes if your follow-up is not going to be as good as it can be and as it needs to be for you to measure the effectiveness of treatment. At the moment I think it is fairly internationally true that, first of all, we don't have very secure measurements of inter-ocular differences that are standardized and that are better than an octave difference between the eyes (which is quite a big difference for acuity between the eyes for young children) up until they can do a crowded letter test or something like that at 4 years. We don't have reliable training of all the people who would do refractions, and we could argue about whether they should be done under cycloplegia or without, or whether they should be done with tropicamide or cyclopentolate, throughout that period of time. So that we've got a lot of questions to answer and a lot of variability in the follow-up system at the moment. From my personal perspective in carrying out the right randomized controlled trial, twice, from 9 months of age, I realize that the follow-up data isn't quite good enough for answering all those questions all the time. I can answer some of the questions about refractive changes, but we can't answer some of the questions on children who developed strabismus and were sent on to a National Health hospital and didn't get followed up for reasons that I don't begin to understand. I have missing data on these children. Now, that may be my problem for not designing the perfect follow-up, but I mean if this is what happens in a good place like Cambridge, how much more common is it everywhere else? So my feelings would really be that we do have to think about what we can do at the moment and where we can go in analysing infant amblyopia if such exists. The trial that we could successfully carry out at the present time, and where we do have adequate measures, would be a trial where we screened a total population of $4\frac{1}{2}$-year-olds for refractive errors and amblyopia, and ran a randomized trial of treatment with occlusion.

Moseley: A request for information. About 5 years ago there was a big group in the States who were trying to put together a functional classification of amblyopia. They published one report in *Transactions of the American Ophthalmological Society.* Whatever happened?

Kiorpes: That's John Flynn's group, and they are in the final stages of publishing all of the psychophysical data. They have vast data on classification, but only on adults.

Part V. Discussion following a review: *Treatment and its Evaluation*, presented by Merrick Moseley

Hess: Perceptual learning is often associated with tasks where multiple cues can be used to solve the task and it takes you some time to get around to learning about what trick to use, so in that respect it's not necessarily a reflection of perceptual plasticity, you know in the sense you are using it.

Moseley: In Levi's paper he does address that issue, he does point that out and concludes that it wasn't a problem in his data.

Hess: Well, I think that sort of (vernier) stimulus may be open to this sort of criticism.

Simons: I'd say about Dennis's study that, as I recall, the learning was very task-specific; indeed, the vertical line didn't generalize to the horizontal line. This aspect is obviously relevant to any practical application. For the two subjects with Snellen acuity improvement, I don't remember if they had been treated before and been on maintenance regimens a couple of times. I would regard the improvements as possibly being, in effect, a repeat maintenance response.

Moseley: I believe they had all been treated.

Hess: What is the status of partial versus total occlusion, is there a consensus on this?

Simons: Some would question whether in reality there are any patients out there that do full time, or whether this is a mass illusion that paediatric ophthalmologists have!

Moseley: Unless you measure compliance in the manner I described, you won't know what is happening!

Simons: The chief appeal of penalization is the phenomenal difference in compliance – near perfect in our and some other studies. Some parents have been known to come back and ask if you can penalize for a little longer to achieve an even better outcome. Now, anybody who prescribes patching would sit there with jaw agape if that were to happen in their clinic!

Atkinson: What is the regimen for penalization?

Simons: There is quite a debate about this. There is a new intermittent regimen in which kids get given a drop, two to three days a week, as opposed to the nominal, so-called full-time, which is supposed to be 7 days a week. But even with the full-time regimen compliance is often less than perfect, so the question is, did anybody ever really do full time? So should the compromise position end up being maybe 4 or 5 days a week?

Moseley: Let's take on a big question . . . what's is actually happening in penalization?

Simons: Well, the mechanism which is traditionally thought to be operative is that you are compromising high frequency spatial frequency responses in the sound eye in order to free up the suppression in the amblyopic eye.

Moseley: . . .but you can still see high spatial frequencies at distance.

Simons: Yes, but since kids' worlds tend to be very near, statistically they tend to be more inclined to look up close.

Doran: There is a dosage regimen in strabismic amblyopia which suggests you progressively defocus the preferred eye until you see a switch in fixation, is that not still valid?

Simons: It turns out to be a hassle to do. The brute force approach of just prescribing the drops and monitoring the result turns out to be, functionally speaking, a close enough approximation.

Doran: Penalization obviously has a differential effect depending on refractive error and whether or not you withdraw the spectacle correction.

Simons: One of the inclusion criteria you have to make is that the child is hypermetropic.

Fielder: I would like to ask the group about the use of controls in RCTs of treatment effectiveness. Whether controls are those that have no intervention at all, or whether spectacles can be considered an adequate control? Does the control have to be an eye that has had no treatment at all?

Doran: From the ethical point of view, or from the point of view of determining the treatment effect?

Fielder: Well obviously ethics is an issue . . .

Clarke: We included a spectacle group in our study because of your work (Moseley *et al.*, 1998) showing that spectacle adaptation did seem to have a treatment effect.

Fielder: The reason we originally did it was to be sure we got a good treatment baseline. The only reason we wanted to study the spectacle issue was so that before we started doing any occlusion we were sure we had a stable baseline of acuity. We had never heard of an RCT at that stage.

Clarke: But you were surprised that a positive treatment effect occurred with spectacles at a stage when conventionally children would have started being patched. What we were anxious to exclude is that we weren't mixing up a treatment effect of spectacles with a treatment effect of patching.

Moseley: I think we appreciate the scientific underpinning of it. But I am just slightly worried that those children would see better if you put their spectacles on them.

Clarke: Well, I think ethics and ethical are very powerful words, so we should be careful how we use them. I don't have any trouble with the ethics of our study. It is deferred treatment in a monitored group with a stopping rule, so we have a get-out clause if children are getting worse: they will fall out of the study. They will still have the opportunity to have treatment if we decide that is what is appropriate at $4-4\frac{1}{2}$ years old, which is the same age they would have received treatment in areas without pre-school vision screening where they would have been screened at school entry. At the end of the day we are talking about amblyopia, and nobody ever died of amblyopia.

Moseley: So you are not worried that these children will be 'bumping into walls', whereas if you just put specs on them they wouldn't?

Clarke: These are children with unilateral visual acuity defects. One of the difficulties I found as an ophthalmologist who's come into this area with no real prior knowledge of screening is that you see a wriggling 3-year-old child who is 6/6 and 6/9, who you refracted to the best of your ability, and you find a dioptre of astigmatism. Now, I did my Fellowship in North America where you correct that, and in retrospect I'm sure I gave a lot of 3-year-olds spectacles who actually didn't really need them.

Fielder: But the trouble is that you've made a massive assumption, and you may be right, I've got no feeling for this. But can we be sure that the visual deficits that you are not correcting, albeit temporarily, are not disabling in any way? For future education?

Clarke: It is a temporary thing.

Atkinson: Do you actually know what their acuity is with refractive correction in place even if you don't give them their spectacles?

Clarke: At the end we do.

Atkinson: So you don't know whether their acuity would have been better with their refractive correction or without?

Clarke: Our trial is not a trial of amblyopia treatment. It is a trial of visual acuity defects that are discovered at pre-school vision screening at the age of 3, so you are quite right, we don't know if some of those children have a refractive error which may or may not have ironed itself out over the year of the course of the trial. The problem about putting them in their specs and then re-testing them at the beginning is that you don't know whether just doing that has had a treatment effect.

Atkinson: So you couldn't say they were truly untreated then?

Clarke: That's right. You can't say at the end that they are truly untreated, because they may have had some treatment by having a month's worth of spectacle wear.

Stewart-Brown: Mike, Merrick was talking about children who were 'bumping into walls'. I don't think they are in the trial, are they?

Clarke: No, no they're not.

Stewart-Brown: It is a terribly important point because they are then asymptomatic: there is no apparent problem with their vision.

Fielder: I saw a child the other day who was 5 or so, 6/24, 6/6, and mum said to me: 'my daughter doesn't use her vision when she wants to do something fine, she has to use her fingers'. She was just an anisometropic amblyope who had been identified quite late, and basically she had some quite significant coordination problems.

Clarke: I think that's unfair, Alistair, that's one case. There are big studies which show no great measurable differences.

Stewart-Brown: Again, Alistair, you may have two separate problems in one child. That's the sort of thing that needs investigating in a bigger study, and one of the ways of doing it is to plug it into the sort of study where you have a no-treatment arm.

Simons: My impression is that the profound difference between strabismic and anisometropic amblyopia hasn't really sunk in, in some quarters.

Stewart-Brown: There is another important difference between the groups. You don't really need to screen for strabismic amblyopes because you should see the strabismus.

Simons: Not true! There's a whole grey area of people who are intermittent, late onset, accommodative; it is not a black and white issue. In congenital ETs, so-called, yes, but beyond that it gets fuzzy, patients with high phorias and so on . . .

Reeves: The outcome comparison between strabismics and anisometropes is confounded by age. It is really interesting to know whether there is really a difference in what is going on, or whether you have just got younger children who are strabismic than you have anisometropic. I don't know of a straight comparison adjusted for age of presentation or age of onset. But going back to perceptual learning, my view of this is that it could be a criterion shift rather than neural plasticity that is occurring. If it were a criterion shift, you would not expect the improvement to be maintained.

Moseley: From the little I've seen of the data, it certainly looks like improvement is maintained over a much longer period than in the pharmacological studies.

Simons: There was a Swedish study in the '60s with 10-year follow-up that reported a finding that I've never seen anybody pick up on which may be central to this issue, and that was that kids with better binocularity tended to stay straighter, setting up a feedback loop situation; less deviation means, presumably, less stimulus for amblyogenic suppression, thus better long-term follow-up results in terms of the amblyopia reduction as well. This presumably contributes in turn to better binocularity so that, again, you have a positive feedback loop situation. In other words, looking at amblyopia by itself in this situation would be to miss an important aspect affecting outcome.

Doran: Coming back to the psychophysics of penalization . . . what do people think about the fact that you thereby maintain alignment and all you apparently subtract is high spatial frequency detail from the visual image? Binocularity seems to be used in rather a loose sense in that case.

Simons: Well, as I understand, and Robert can correct me on this, both fusion and stereopsis – the fundamental mechanisms – are active at surprisingly low spatial frequencies, so you are legitimately maintaining the binocular channel in penalization.

Hess: Well, it would certainly affect stereoacuity, but binocular function in general would still be operative in the low spatial frequency range.

Simons: I think the reason the question was raised as to whether binocularity was a legitimate argument to make is because one of penalization's claims to fame is that it keeps binocularity intact, and if binocularity is based on low spatial frequencies then it's really intact and that's a plus.

Hess: Well, that sounds reasonable. If you lose high spatial frequencies, your stereoacuity will be reduced. But for spatially broadband stimuli like that of the real world there should be ample stimulation of low spatial frequency disparity sensitive mechanisms. What you are really doing is reducing the range over which disparity information operates, thus retaining a substantial amount of binocular function.

Atkinson: So it's just giving a reduced contrast.

Hess: That's true, but only for narrowband stimuli such as gratings. For broadband stimuli, there is change in the shape of the spectrum and this I think will be a more important effect for everyday images.

Part VI. Discussion following a review: *Disability*, presented by Alistair Fielder

Simons: Cynthia Owsley, working at the geriatric end of the age spectrum, has shown that individuals with what she terms a restricted 'useful field of view' show a much higher traffic accident rate. Well, extrapolating that to the paediatric age range, I think a useful initial index of disability would be a morbidity index; nothing to do with the eyes *per se* but simply injury rate. I would even hypothesize a laterality effect – a right-eyed amblyope having more injuries on their right arm or on the right side of their left arm and so on.

Doran: Children these days are rather more involved with video-interactive experiences. Isn't this an ideal scenario to test these questions (on disability)?

Fielder: Perhaps amblyopic children tend *not* to play video games.

Blakemore: Video games are two-dimensional, with a relatively small visual display. I'm not sure that they would provide the right kind of stimulus.

Simons: Comparing injury rates passes your key tabloid headline test – 'Amblyopic Kids Get Hurt More!'. That is something that everybody understands.

Atkinson: But not because they are amblyopic. It may not be that their amblyopia has led to their clumsiness.

Stewart-Brown: It could be their squint.

Atkinson: It may not be their squint which has led to their clumsiness.

Kiorpes: But if you have a high enough incidence of clumsiness you can start to draw some correlations.

Stewart-Brown: But you can't assume that treating the amblyopia is going to cure the clumsiness unless you understand the causality.

Atkinson: I've done the Goodale experiment on babies, comparing monocular and binocular vision, and I've also done it on clinical populations who were not strabismic. If you occlude one eye in normal young babies they go to a reach that is a more primitive, younger reach, and they look more developmentally delayed monocularly; these are babies that have stereopsis so they are using stereopsis normally for reaching. Now I can test a group of clinical children who don't squint and who don't have amblyopia and I can test the same group who do squint and do have amblyopia, and I can find the same level of problem in delayed reaching and grasping in those two groups, and what that tells me is that there isn't necessarily a causal link but there is a correlational link, so you can use amblyopia to pick up soft signs of other problems.

Blakemore: Perhaps what I have to say is naïve, but if you just cover one eye, the most immediate and obvious effects are: (1) a reduction of the total width of the visual field by nearly 20 degrees, which is likely to interfere with the analysis of optic flow and therefore with driving, and (2) total loss of stereopsis, which is very likely to compromise fine motor control. Now, I suppose that practice could help to overcome some of the disadvantages of working with one eye, but not all of them. Finally, in the case of uncorrected or inadequately corrected squint, by far the biggest disability the child suffers is one of cosmetic appearance, which can be a severe social handicap.

Stewart-Brown: The issue about squints is very, very important, and I'm sure you are absolutely right, but it is totally different from the treatment of amblyopia and the thing about the loss of one eye – absolutely true when you have absolute loss of vision, but 80 per cent of the amblyopes who go through treatment programmes at the moment have a visual loss less than 6/36. We are not talking about a blind eye, we're talking about an eye with reduced vision.

Blakemore: But measurement of visual acuity through the amblyopic eye alone may not provide a full account of its contribution to normal vision, nor of the patient's visual problems. For instance, when both eyes are open, active suppression of the amblyopic eye may render it virtually blind.

Simons: That is a very critical point. Amblyopia is measured clinically with the other eye closed, and there have been a few vectorgraphic studies that demonstrate that the functional loss in the amblyopic eye typically drops off appreciably further under two-eyed viewing conditions. This additional suppression-based loss is not convenient to measure clinically, however, and the result is a classic demonstration of how a measurement has determined a concept, i.e. the definition of amblyopic deficit level is based on a monocular acuity measure that does not in fact reflect the full deficit under normal binocular viewing conditions.

Fielder: Remember of course the effect of age. Disability may appear at different ages, so one has to be very careful of measuring at one particular age and then extrapolating to other ages. We haven't mentioned visual information processing tasks, such as speed of reading.

Simons: The injury index approach would fit right in with the hypothesized defects in visual information processing. Consider a moving tool coming up toward your face . . . Now this is not going to be easy to measure, and I don't know if this kind of thing has ever been quantitatively characterized. But what is crucial is that it doesn't seem to matter whether you use one eye or two eyes in many perceptual judgements, but what I bet does get reduced a lot in the monocular condition is the 'information processing' speed with which you can make accurate judgement of depth. So when you are navigating through a complex visual world, the speed at which an amblyope can make these judgements will be much reduced.

Fielder: But I thought Goodale looked at that and didn't find a difference if head movements were allowed.

Clarke: In the real world, there are a number of amblyopic sportsmen who function well.

Blakemore: But catching a moving object, as in many sports, depends essentially on a two-dimensional estimate of the angular separation between the object and the body, and an estimate of the time-to-contact. Most sports do not depend critically on stereopsis (fine relative depth discrimination). Surely, the extraordinary acuity of stereopsis is most important when we use our hands for fine tasks. Ask an amblyope to thread a needle . . . they may achieve it, but with difficulty, using a strategy quite different from those of us lucky enough to have stereopsis.

Fielder: So you wouldn't have your cataract removed by an amblyopic eye surgeon?!

Stewart-Brown: But it shouldn't be that difficult to find all these things, and then when you have a child in the clinic with the parent you can say to the parent what it is they're not going to be able to do if you are not going to patch or treat them. Everybody is coming up with ideas, all of which are perfectly valid and plausible, and yet what I am saying is that we need to do the research to document how common these things are and how much of a hassle it is to people. Everything we are saying seems to support the idea that it would be a good idea to tease this out as opposed to us all sitting here disagreeing.

Harrad: A couple of points on disability. There are obviously a number of jobs that you can't do. You mentioned eye surgery as one of them, but obviously the armed forces is another, and the police. You can't be a guard on a train unless you've got better than 6/18 vision in both eyes, and you can't drive an HGV unless you have good vision in both eyes. If you are from a certain part of the country, and you have certain employment prospects, there are a significant number of occupations that won't be open to you if you are moderately amblyopic or worse.

Fielder: That is true, but of course it's historical rather than evidence-based.

Clarke: I wouldn't want my cataract done by a uniocular ophthalmologist either, but there is a chap in the States who defends, in a court of law, physicians who are told they cannot enter ophthalmology training programmes.

Fielder: I retrospectively know that I have had several amblyopic trainees working for me in the past.

Stewart-Brown: I think it would be perfectly reasonable for somebody to bring a case against a train operating company for unequal employment opportunities because there is absolutely no evidence that you can't do the job with amblyopia and 6/18 acuity. There is reasonable evidence that you can fly perfectly well with it, so the fact that occupational health doctors in the past have made silly judgements doesn't mean to say that we should be sorting out kids now to sort out a problem that doctors have created.

Harrad: Well, this is how the law stands in this country at the moment.

Stewart-Brown: Well we *should* challenge it.

Doran: If you are looking for the evidence, would you find it in probability or would you exclude it using 'black swan' as the exception to the rule? Popper used this metaphor in discussing how scientific theory should be phrased, i.e. 'All swans are white' is a closed hypothesis which is liable to challenge the discovery of a black swan. A better hypothesis would be in the negative, i.e. 'not all swans are white'. So possibly 'not all amblyopes are clumsy'; 'not all amblyopes make inept eye surgeons'?. So if you found a particular eye surgeon with very dense amblyopia in one eye but who is nonetheless an excellent surgeon, would you then extrapolate that case to all cases, or would you say on average amblyopes with acuity worse than 6/24 in their amblyopic eye are not so good at being eye surgeons, so therefore in general you were going to make this an entry criteria?

Stewart-Brown: Well I think if you identify the outcomes first of all, i.e. good at surgery, bad at surgery, you can then do some sort of population study where you decide that, say, 20 per cent of them are good at it and 80 per cent of them are bad at it, or the other way round, at which point you can start making some sort of judgement. But first of all you have got to decide if it's threading needles, which I think is very likely to be an issue, or what sort of tasks that people seem to have difficulty with. One of the difficulties, if you go and talk to people, which is what we've started to do, is that it is jolly difficult to perceive you've got a problem with something you've never been able to do in any other way. That seems to be the intellectual conundrum with amblyopia: you are trying to ask people to tell you that they have difficulty with a task that they have managed to learn how to do, but they've never done it the easy way because they've never had that ability.

Fielder: This is akin to the totally blind person who says 'I'm jolly lucky because I've been blind since birth'. What they really mean is that they have no concept of what it is like to be any other way.

Blakemore: Many of these concerns resonate with me. Much clinical attention in this country is directed at providing generally unpalatable forms of treatment, with little prospect of long-term remediation, to children who are already fairly well adapted to their deficiencies. Children hate wearing patches and often don't comply, and parents are frequently disappointed with the outcome. However, what this says to me is not that we should give up completely and pretend there isn't a problem, but that we should be more radical in our strategy for tackling what is, after all, the commonest cause of referral of young people to ophthalmologists. In my opinion, we should be aiming at prevention or very early treatment, when the visual system is still highly 'plastic' and when we know from both animal studies and work on babies that remarkable and enduring results can be achieved. Children who lose their hearing completely in one ear actually learn to do pretty well with their one remaining ear; people who lose a leg can, with an appropriate prosthesis, make remarkable progress. But this doesn't mean that we should be unconcerned about the loss of an ear or a leg. We should concentrate, wherever possible, on prevention.

Fielder: Well, I would think that there is no one in the room who would disagree with that.

Simons: Well I would disagree with one thing. If penalization is as good as patching for at least moderate amblyopia, which I am virtually convinced that it is, then that completely eliminates the compliance problem.

Fielder: This takes us back to our spectacle adaptation study where if you do not start occlusion until you have improved acuity as much as you can with spectacles you are more likely to get better compliance, because vision in the amblyopic eye is better than had you started occlusion immediately.

Stewart-Brown: There are two aspects to the discomfort of being treated. One is the physical patch, which children hate, and having it taken on and off, which they hate, and the other one is having your vision impaired when you have a good eye, and presumably you get that with penalization. So the only thing that's better with penalization is you don't have the horrible piece of plaster coming on and off. Is that right?

Simons: Well, it does blur vision, although you have more or less normal vision at distance and, again, if you start early enough children will accept this because it becomes the norm for them. If you wait until school age it becomes a problem: mum's not going to put up with her child doing badly in school, and there will be a lack of compliance for social and academic reasons. The real punch line in this whole thing for me is very political and not only in the UK and it gets my steam pressure right up there . . . paediatrics across the board just does not get the funding it deserves relative to older age groups, and I think this has a lot to do with the age of MPs and Congressmen. I have heard it said in this country that amblyopia research will not get the funding it deserves until you have a royal baby with strabismus!

Harrad: Colin talked about losing an ear, losing a leg, but the fact is that the parents of straight-eyed amblyopes are not aware of there being any problem. Parents have to look after them and decide for them on their behalf what treatment they should have. I see a number of patients every year who have been seen elsewhere who come to me for a second opinion. The child is 7 or 8 and has 6/36 to 6/60 vision in one eye due to undiagnosed anisometropic amblyopia. These parents are absolutely furious. This is a child who is in effect nearly blind in one eye. Somebody has missed it, two people have missed it, three people have missed it, and the parents are very upset and angry and are often threatening to sue. They feel that this child, that they thought they were looking after properly, has been let down at various stages by various people, and it is difficult for me to convey the degree of indignation and distress that these parents bring along when they come and see me, and that just gives me an idea of the kind of interest and energy parents are going to have in having their child treated. Parents have an idea that their child is going to be perfect, they want their child to be perfect, and they have a right for their child to be perfect, and I think that these people out there want us to provide these perfect children for them, and screening seems to me to be a jolly good way of going about doing this. I think that when we are assessing disability, the parent's idea of the child's disability, their concern for the child's future, and their need to have a 'whole child' are important elements that don't seem to have been discussed very much up until now.

Atkinson: I support that very strongly.

Vital-Durand: I think this is a very important issue.

Fielder: We are not talking about a child, are we, we are talking about a family.

Vital-Durand: When you talk to people who have lived with a single eye for 80 years you will find that they don't say they spent their time asking a psychiatrist for help, but they may say they had a life of anxiety about losing their single good eye . . . I am surprised that so much emphasis has been put on screening at $3\frac{1}{2}$ years and not earlier. I would agree that treatment at $3\frac{1}{2}$ years of age will allow a recovery of the amblyopic eye, but at a high price in terms of length of occlusion regimen. Why not have a first check at 9 months when everything is easy, including patching compliance. This procedure would not exclude a further screening at $3\frac{1}{2}$ years to catch the misses and the newly developed amblyopia. This would not leave many adults with an amblyopia!

Stewart-Brown: I went out to talk to people with amblyopia with one of my researchers. We didn't do a huge sample, but we asked the ophthalmologist to refer every person with amblyopia they came across, child, adult, parent, if we could talk to them about what their amblyopia had done to them, how it had affected them, and they did not tell us what you are saying they all feel.

Vital-Durand: Well, I am surprised at that. It does not fit with our observations.

Stewart-Brown: This was a very sensitive qualitative researcher, and all the evidence suggests that people talk to qualitative researchers more than they do to their doctors. If they had something about which they are as distressed as you feel, and it was common, we would have expected to see it in that study. What I am saying is, it may happen and we didn't have anything like the numbers to rule it out, but the people we were talking to were not terribly distressed by their amblyopia.

Vital-Durand: Well, I'm surprised at that.

Woodruff: I think the extent to which the child has difficulty with amblyopia is important, but you dismissed rather quickly the disability the patient may develop from losing the eye in later life. I suspect you dismissed this because Tomilla and Tarkinen's much quoted paper on this subject is hopelessly inadequate. However, there are other sources of information. First of all, Jugnoo Rahi's survey of ophthalmologists in the UK asking them to report loss of the good eye in amblyopes will give us a much better idea of the size of the problems. Secondly, you can also get some information by knowing about the prevalence of unilateral visual loss. While we have much less information about the prevalence of unilateral visual loss than bilateral visual loss, there is some data on this. A study of a rural Appalachian community in Mud River Creek Valley found that 5.4 per cent of the population over the age of 40 years had vision in one eye reduced to less than 6/18. So in this community the risk for an amblyope of having unilateral visual loss in the other eye would have been 2.7 per cent. In this community, 17 per cent of patients over the age of 80 years had unilateral visual loss, suggesting that in this community an amblyope who reached his 80s would have an approximately 7.5 per cent chance of having unilateral visual loss in the non-amblyopic eye and bitterly regretting he had amblyopia.

Rahi: (to Harrad) A comment on screening. For every parent that comes to you very upset that their child has not been diagnosed, there may be three who didn't attend their screening examination and a further two who did not follow-up after their first examination, and that is the reality of it. The best screening programmes that exist in most places have attendance rates of 70 per cent, and then compliance after that with treatment falls off, so there is a message in that. The reality of it is that you instigate a service in a district, the right screeners doing the examination at the right time and all the rest of it, and yet people don't turn up and they don't come back, and that is because they have other problems to deal with. They don't necessarily see the amblyopia of their child as a major problem, and it is the whole person you are dealing with and the whole family who may well have other problems. This is the problem. We assume that parents are all are very upset about this, but they may not be as upset as we think.

Doran: The reason why intervening younger doesn't work is that some anisometropes lose there anisometropia in their very early years and others acquire an anisometropia, and that is why Abrahamsson and colleagues suggest an age between 3 and 4. But there is another reason, the case who came to see Richard Harrad at age of 7 with marked anisometropic amblyopia may in fact have posterior lenticonus as an acquired lesion even later than 4 years of age causing amblyopia, so my main thesis here is that we cannot assume in advance what the aetiology and/or the time scale and/or the severity of the amblyopia might be simply on the basis of age.

Williams: A lot of what's been said exemplifies our need to know about the relevance of visual functions to other skills such as information processing, for amblyopes and for individuals with no visual problems. If deficits in visual abilities are correlated with deficits in other skills, then those skills should be considered as outcomes in trials of early intervention for amblyopia in order to explore whether there is evidence of a causal relationship. Any such evidence would be very important in debates about treatment or screening for amblyopia.

Atkinson: I would like to support Colin's comments, which were that we should be more hopeful in thinking about prevention and early prevention rather than just the consequences. We need to think about the consequences, but we desperately need to think about better studies done earlier, which are the kinds of trial which we have been trying to do, and we need to think about that very seriously because at the moment we are held up for lack of information as to whether these are correlations or causally related in a lot of children.

Stewart-Brown: (to Fielder) I think that if you are going to argue the case that we should have screening programmes universally in place in child health, you would need the data as to what the problem causes later on in order to make the economic argument in the face of other screening programmes.

Atkinson: And that is exactly what we are trying to do, and there are lots of points to be made not just to do with the screening but with the number of people available for doing good follow-up and collecting the data and analysing the data properly. That lack is quite apparent to me now in some areas. It is really in terms of very early prevention of amblyopia where we could be most effective, and to carry out these trials successfully we need to know the precursors of amblyopia.

Fielder: Because almost certainly you would end up treating a lot of children who didn't need it, wouldn't you?

Atkinson: You have got to find that out, before you can actually decide which are the relevant groups to treat.

REFERENCES

Jacobs, D. S. and Blakemore, C. (1988). Factors limiting the postnatal development of visual acuity in the monkey. *Vision Res.*, **28**, 947–58.

Kiorpes, L., Kiper, D. C., O'Keefe, L. P. *et al.* (1998). Neuronal correlates of amblyopia in the visual cortex of macaque monkeys with experimental strabismus and anisometropia. *J. Neurosci.*, **18**, 6411–24.

Kubova, Z., Kuba, M., Juran, J. and Blakemore, C. (1996). Is the motion system relatively spared in amblyopia? Evidence from cortical evoked responses. *Vision Res.*, **36**, 181–90.

Moseley, M. J., Neufeld, M. and Fielder, A. R. (1998). Treatment of amblyopia by spectacles. *Invest. Ophthalmol. Vis. Sci.*, **39**, S332.

Simons, K. and Preslan, M. (1999). Natural history of amblyopia due to lack of compliance. *Br. J. Ophthalmol.*, **83**, 582–7.

Index

RETURN TO: **OPTOMETRY LIBRARY**
490 Minor Hall • 642-1020

LOAN PERIOD	1	2	3
1 MONTH	4	5	6

All books may be recalled after 7 days.
Renewals may be requested by phone or, using GLADIS,
type **inv** followed by your patron ID number.

DUE AS STAMPED BELOW.

This book will be held in OPTOMETRY LIBRARY until ___ AUG 2 2 2002	
JUL 1 0 2004	
OCT 1 0 2004	
MAY – 8 2005	
JUL 2 2 2005	
OCT 2 1 2005	
DEC 1 4 2006	
AUG 2 5 2010	

FORM NO. DD 17
1M 3-01

UNIVERSITY OF CALIFORNIA, BERKELEY
Berkeley, California 94720–6000